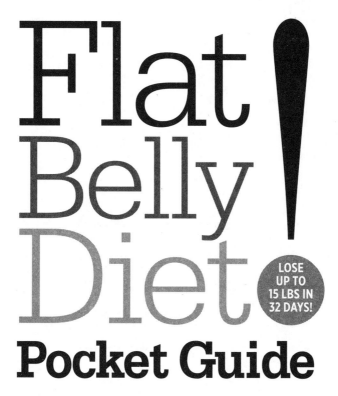

Flat Belly Diet!

LOSE UP TO 15 LBS IN 32 DAYS!

Pocket Guide

Introducing the EASIEST, BUDGET-MAXIMIZING Eating Plan Yet!

LIZ VACCARIELLO, Editor-in-Chief of **Prevention**.
Coauthor of the *New York Times* best-selling diet

© 2009 by Rodale, Inc.

Rodale books may be purchased for business or promotional use or for special sales. For information, please write to:
Special Markets Department, Rodale Inc.,
733 Third Avenue, New York, NY 10017

Printed in the United States of America
Rodale Inc. makes every effort to use acid-free ♾, recycled paper ♻.

Book design by Jill Armus and Christina Gaugler

Library of Congress Cataloging-in-Publication Data is on file with the publisher.

ISBN 13: 978-1-60529-650-0
ISBN 10: 1-60529-650-3

Distributed to the trade by Macmillan

6   8   10   9   7   5   hardcover

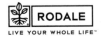

We inspire and enable people to improve their lives and the world around them

For more of our products visit **rodalestore.com** or call 800-848-4735

CONTENTS

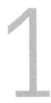
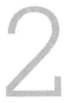
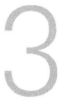
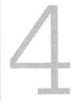

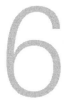

INTRODUCTION

I **don't know anyone who doesn't want a flat belly.** I have friends who moan about their post-baby bulge. I have colleagues who are dumbfounded by their 40-plus pooch. And I have neighbors who point guiltily to the "beer belly" that's getting rounder, hanging lower over the belt buckle. Even my lean (lucky) friends bemoan their propensity to bloat.

When *Prevention* magazine polled Americans about the body part they most wanted to change, an incredible 67 percent said their belly. It's clear we're craving a solution to belly fat. And no wonder. Countless public health authorities continue to remind us that belly fat is the most dangerous fat you can have on your body. Even small excess amounts of it can increase your risk of high blood pressure, heart disease, diabetes, dementia, and breast cancer. The combination of these two factors (health first, vanity second) is why I wanted to write the *Flat Belly Diet!* **I wanted to find the absolute best way to permanently lose belly fat.**

But I didn't just want to construct a diet and name it the *Flat Belly Diet*. I had always heard it was impossible to spot reduce, but then *Prevention*'s nutrition director came into my office with some exciting new research that showed there was a way to eat that might affect the belly specifically! The study was published in the journal *Diabetes Care*, and it showed that eating a diet high in monounsaturated fatty acids—or MUFAs (pronounced MOO-fahs)—could help prevent the accumulation of belly fat, or more specifically, the visceral fat that we've been told to be so concerned about. MUFAs are found in foods like nuts, seeds, avocados, and olive oil, and this is the only diet that features a precise serving of these healthful, filling foods in every meal you eat.

On the *Flat Belly Diet*, you'll begin with the 4-Day Anti-Bloat Jump-start. This part of the diet will leave you, on average, 4 pounds lighter and at least 1 inch smaller around the waist, not to mention more confident and motivated! It's a very prescriptive phase of the *Flat Belly Diet* that enables you to flush out excess fluid. The success you will achieve during this short time frame will spark your commitment to the entire program. The regular eating plan lasts a minimum of 28 days. This is where MUFAs take center stage, and it's where the real fat loss begins. Each meal and each snack features a MUFA-rich food such as crunchy nuts, creamy avocado, or flavorful dark chocolate.

The positive response to the *Flat Belly Diet* has exceeded my wildest expectations. I've heard from literally thousands of *Flat Belly Diet*ers thanking us for this plan. We followed nine of them in our test panel. One woman, Mary Anne Speshok, lost 15 pounds and 10 inches in just 32 days—and loved the food so much she continued the plan to lose a total of 49 pounds in 5 months! Although not everyone will see the same results, each of our testers was thrilled to see their bellies shrink—and, in many cases, their blood pressure and cholesterol numbers improve as well.

Still, there's nothing like scientific proof to go along with real-world success, so in the summer of 2008, we commissioned the scientists at Yale University–Griffin Hospital to study the 28-day plan's effect on visceral fat. This independent study consisted of nine female participants, all overweight or obese at the start. Scientists weighed them, measured their waistlines, took their blood, and ran a battery of baseline tests to determine starting levels of cholesterol, inflammation, and other important health markers. Then each woman was put through an MRI scan, so the researchers could get an internal view of her belly fat.

After 28 days on the *Flat Belly Diet*, the women were fully screened again, and the results, my friends, astounded us.

In this small but significant study, the *Flat Belly Diet* reduced visceral fat—the dangerous belly fat—by an average of 33 percent in just 4 weeks. It also improved nearly every major health marker, lowering total cholesterol by an average of 21 points and reducing biomarkers for insulin resistance and inflammation. Participants lost, on average, 8.4 pounds and 1.6 inches off the waist. You can find more details on the study at prevention.com/flatbellymri. Said David L. Katz, MD, director of the Yale Prevention Research Center, who helped oversee the research, "If the plan were sustained, these women would be at reduced risk for heart disease, diabetes, cancer, you name it. Basically, the diet kicked butt—or, perhaps more appropriately in this case, belly!"

With this Pocket Guide, the *Flat Belly Diet* is easier to follow than ever. In letters and e-mails and on flatbellydiet.com, you've asked for more Quick-and-Easy Meal solutions, more Restaurant Rescues, and more guidance on how to stick with the *Flat Belly Diet* when you're on the go. I enlisted the help of Tracy Gensler, MS, RD, and Samina Riaz, RD, who work with the thousands of members of flatbellydiet.com, to put together a straightforward sample eating plan for the 4-Day Anti-Bloat Jumpstart and the full 28 days of the *Flat Belly Diet*. Their meals are balanced, fast, tasty, economical, and effortless to create.

With Your Ultimate 28-Day Eating Plan, plus tools to make smart eating choices wherever you are, this Pocket Guide is our answer to your questions about how to make the *Flat Belly Diet* a permanent, portable part of your life. I'm thrilled to make this diet accessible to people like you, busy people who care about their health and want the most simple and the most realistic plan. I like to think of this Pocket Guide as the no-brainer *Flat Belly Diet!* If you're eating the *Flat Belly* way already, this guide will help you continue to get results. If you aren't, here's an easy way to try it out.

Now, let's get ready to lose that belly fat!

1.

HOW TO USE
THIS GUIDE

If you've read the *Flat Belly Diet!*, you already know how easy the plan is. Just follow three simple rules and you're well on your way to a trimmer tummy, right? But if, like most women we know, you're juggling work, family, and myriad other responsibilities, even that can sometimes be a challenge. Enter the *Flat Belly Diet! Pocket Guide*.

You don't even need to read through this whole book to get started. Just flip straight to the section that interests you now. If you want a quick overview, Chapter 2, The *Flat Belly Diet* at a Glance, gives you a summary of the plan.

If you want to try the 4-Day Anti-Bloat Jumpstart, start with Chapter 3. The jumpstart isn't necessary to burn belly fat—since it contains no recommended amount of MUFAs—but most people have found that it really helps them get in the habit of eating four meals a day, every 4 hours. Plus, of course, they love that it helps them drop pounds and inches almost instantly!

If you want to learn how to create your own *Flat Belly Diet* meals, Chapter 4 offers a MUFA Meal Maker Guide that explains how to assemble quick and tasty meals with the right ratio of MUFAs to other foods. With tips on how to shop for, store, and use MUFAs and other building blocks of the diet (such as lean protein, dairy, fruits and vegetables, and whole grains), this chapter gives you all the tools you need to understand how this diet works.

If you want to head straight to the supermarket to get started (you don't even need to stop and figure out your shopping list, since we've done that for you!), Chapter 5 lays out Your Ultimate 28-Day Eating Plan and takes the guesswork out of the question *What do I eat next?* We carefully designed the meal plan and grocery lists to maximize your shopping dollar—no wasted leftover portions of foods you'd love to eat but can't. We've also chosen to feature a variety of belly-shrinking MUFAs. All of the meals take less than 20 minutes to prepare, and each is filling and delicious. Plus, most of the meals are portable, so you can easily take them with you if you're on the go.

If you want to customize the 28-day eating plan to better suit your tastes, you'll find 30 additional Quick-and-Easy Meals and Snack Packs in Chapter 6—simply substitute one meal for any other on the plan when you want a little variety. Share your favorites with your fellow *Flat Belly Diet*ers on flatbellydiet.com.

If you're at home, our *Flat Belly Diet* Pantry (in Chapter 4) and *Flat Belly Diet*–Friendly Products (in Chapter 7) will help you whip up meals quickly.

If you're concerned about how to stick to the plan when you're traveling, dining out, or just running errands, we've got you covered with our Restaurant Rescue and Best Meal Choices (in Chapter 7) in the airport, at the movies, or anywhere else you may go.

You'll also find quick reference lists with serving sizes and calorie counts at the end of the book to make it easy for you to calculate how much of each type of food you need for each meal. Use our quick conversion chart to decode nutrition labels and measure your servings. And throughout the book, you'll find fast, healthy eating tips and answers to questions frequently asked on flatbellydiet.com about how to adapt the diet to special needs and tastes.

As you can see, I've designed this guide to give you just the basics so that you can make the *Flat Belly Diet* work for you. Keep this powerful little book on hand to provide instant answers about what to eat when you're at the supermarket, out with friends, or anywhere else. Now it's time to get started!

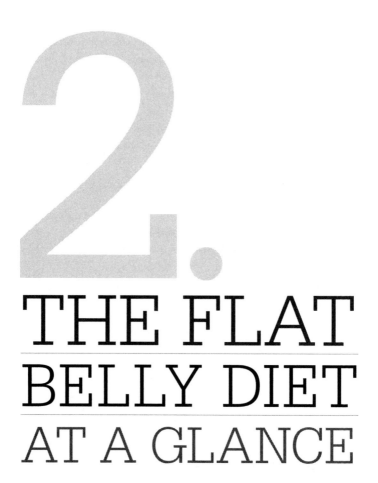

2.

THE FLAT BELLY DIET AT A GLANCE

Prevention readers know a good diet from a fad. They tell me month after month that they like simple instructions, strategies inspired by science, and plans that make logical sense. Most important, they want a diet that will make them healthy and infuse them with energy. That's why I made sure the *Flat Belly Diet* was designed by a registered dietitian with more than 15 years of experience helping people change their bodies and their lives with food. Any diet that contains fewer calories than you're used to eating will help you lose weight, but few weight loss diets actually teach you how to eat to lose pounds *and* maximize your health for life. Here's what makes the *Flat Belly Diet* different.

○ **It's packed with healthful foods.** I've heard that "the hottest thing in Hollywood" is a diet that's composed almost entirely of maple syrup, cayenne pepper, and lemon juice. Does this sound healthy to you? The *Flat Belly Diet* is loaded with foods you know are good for you: vegetables, fruits, whole grains, lean proteins— and of course the all-healthy MUFAs. It's the combination of these foods that makes the *Flat Belly Diet* so tremendously beneficial to your health and well-being.

○ **It's calorie controlled, not low calorie.** A registered dietitian designed the *Flat Belly Diet* to provide approximately 1,600 calories a day (which is the amount the average woman over the age of 40 needs to maintain a healthy weight), so it's by no means a starvation diet. (The online service at flatbellydiet.com allows women *and men* to tailor the *Flat Belly Diet* to different calorie levels, suiting your age, gender, and activity level.) Even better, the plan is divided into four meals per day, and you're required to eat every 4 hours. Each meal provides about 400 calories, and I guarantee you will be pleasantly surprised by how much food this actually is. (Some of the original testers never got used to how filling the breakfasts were!) By spacing out your eating times, you ensure that you never feel hungry. Ever.

○ **It's delicious!** Get ready for "diet food" that you will actually look forward to eating. Peanut butter? Guacamole? Chocolate? Weight loss? Yes indeed. Simply said, *Prevention* readers love the MUFA-rich meals! I have had hundreds of letters from satisfied *Flat Belly Diet*ers thanking us for giving them a way to eat that embraces their favorite foods.

○ **It's refreshingly easy.** Since every meal is nutritionally well balanced and provides roughly the same number of calories, it's simple to swap out meals. Plus, we provide the calorie count for every component of the meal, so swapping individual foods is a no-brainer. Even dining out is easy; simply select the *Flat Belly Diet*-friendly menu picks from the Restaurant Rescue on page 113.

A lot of people who read about the *Flat Belly Diet* on the Web or in the newspaper try to make up their own version of the plan. They might think that adding a dash of olive oil here or a slice of avocado there will somehow magically make them slim. Incorporating these healthy foods even when you're not trying to lose weight is a smart idea, but remember that MUFAs are calorie dense. If you want to lose belly fat, you must follow the *Flat Belly Diet* rules.

RULE #1: STICK TO 400 CALORIES PER MEAL.

Every *Flat Belly Diet* meal and snack contains a MUFA-rich food plus other wholesome foods to total about 400 calories per meal. It's not necessary to make sure every meal is exactly 400 calories, but it is important that, over the course of a day, you get about 1,600 calories. If one meal is a bit over 400, make the next a bit under 400 and so on.

RULE #2: NEVER GO MORE THAN 4 HOURS WITHOUT EATING.

I don't have to tell you that a diet won't work if it makes you feel hungry or tired. That's why on the *Flat Belly Diet* I ask that you eat every 4 hours. This should help you feel fueled and energized, prevent you from feeling hungry, hold cravings at bay, and keep your metabolism revved up, energized, and burning calories throughout the day.

RULE #3: EAT A MUFA AT EVERY MEAL.

Monounsaturated fatty acids, or MUFAs, are the healthy oils found in many plant foods. They are delicious and packed with nutrients, and they fill you up fast (and keep you full longer). You'll find one full MUFA serving in each meal or snack of Your Ultimate 28-Day Eating Plan (page 47). Learn the five categories of MUFAs:

1. Oils

2. Nuts and seeds

3. Avocados

4. Olives

5. Dark chocolate

Later in this guide, you'll get acquainted with the full MUFA list (Your MUFA Serving Chart, page 132) and find out ways to use the MUFAs (How to Shop for, Store, and Use MUFAs, page 24).

The foundation of the *Flat Belly Diet* is the Mediterranean style of eating, the gold standard of nutrition for optimal health and disease prevention. That's why the food lists are limited to whole foods or very minimally processed foods that are naturally rich in plant-based anti-oxidants, fiber, and other healthful nutrients. MUFAs serve "double duty" so to speak. They fight belly fat (as well as heart disease, type 2 diabetes, high blood pressure, and cancer), and their antioxidants and other natural substances (such as resveratrol in nuts and dark choco-late, oleocanthal in olive oil, beta-sitosterol in avocado, etc.) protect your health in other ways, too!

The *Flat Belly Diet* is made up of two parts—the 4-Day Anti-Bloat Jumpstart and Your Ultimate 28-Day Eating Plan. The 4-day jump-start is specifically designed to target belly bloat and water retention, whereas the 28-day plan featuring MUFA-rich foods is designed to help reduce belly and overall body fat.

3.

THE 4-DAY ANTI-BLOAT JUMPSTART

The goal of the jumpstart is to help you reduce or eliminate bloating and the sluggishness that accompanies it. It's important to keep in mind that the results of the jumpstart are highly dependent on your habits before you started. But many *Flat Belly Diet*ers reported feeling energized after the jumpstart and found it a great transition (physically and mentally) to the regular plan.

THE FOUR BAD GUYS OF BLOAT

Here are four lifestyle factors that can influence how prone you are to bloating or fluid retention.

1. **Stress.** A stressful event triggers hormone fluctuations that raise blood pressure and divert blood to your extremities, causing your digestive system to slow down. This can leave that last meal sitting around in your intestine a little longer, causing bloat.

2. **Lack of fluid.** It's true that you need about 8 glasses of water a day. Drinking water and eating "watery" foods such as greens, melon, and other fruits and vegetables guard against water retention and constipation, which can cause bloating.

3. **Lack of sleep.** Your nervous system depends on adequate sleep. Too little sleep disrupts the intricate workings of this system, which controls the rhythmic contractions of your GI tract and helps keep things humming along.

4. **Air travel.** The average plane maintains cabin pressure equal to 5,000 to 8,000 feet above sea level in order to provide a comfortable atmosphere for the passengers. At that altitude, free air in the body cavities tends to expand by around 25 percent. Pressure changes also increase the production of gases in your digestive system. As the

WHERE'S THE MUFA?

Since the jumpstart attacks belly bloat and water retention, the foods selected during these 4 days are chosen based on their ability to prevent or reduce bloating. In other words, any foods you see that serve as MUFAs during the regular plan, such as olive oil, are only included during the jumpstart for their ability to help with bloating. There is not a "*MUFA at every meal*" during the jumpstart phase.

pressure in the cabin drops, the air in your intestines expands, causing bloating and discomfort. Cabin pressurization is also responsible for increased water retention because it impacts your body's natural fluid balance. Add in the dehydration caused by recirculated air, and those bloat miles add up. Before and during your flight, drink as much water as possible and walk around as often as possible during the flight.

JUMPSTART BASICS

Follow the 4-Day meal plan exactly.

This includes four smaller meals, one of which is a refreshing, bloat-blasting smoothie. You'll notice that there are generally healthy foods, such as raw vegetables and citrus fruits, that we ask you to avoid during the 4-day jumpstart. These foods provide great nutritional value, but can contribute to bloat because of their bulk and acidity. So, while we don't want you to shun these foods forever (in fact, you'll see many of them appear in your 28-day eating plan), we've banned them from your diet for these 4 days to focus on reducing your belly bloat. Instead, we carefully chose foods that deliver a lot of nutritional and bloat-free bang for your buck *and* that need no added salt or condiments to taste good, so you won't be tempted to reach for potential bloat promoters.

THE RIGHT WAY TO HYDRATE

Limit water intake to a little over 2 liters, or up to 10 (8-ounce) glasses, per day. Your kidneys do a good job of filtering excess water, but more than this is generally not needed for nonactive hours. You'll see that this is the amount of Sassy Water we ask you to drink each day during the 4-day jumpstart. We encourage you to keep that up during the 28-day eating plan, as well.

That being said, if there are foods on the 4-day jumpstart that you're allergic to, we have provided a list of approved substitutes. Again, please stick to these substitutes, which were carefully chosen to give you balanced nutrition without promoting bloat.

Eat four 300-calorie meals a day.

The 4-day jumpstart includes fewer calories—about 1,200 daily—than you'll be eating on the rest of the *Flat Belly Diet*, which allows about 1,600 per day. Eating less for these 4 days reduces the amount of food in your GI tract at any one time, cuts back on the release of stomach acids, and gets your body used to a four-meal-a-day schedule.

Drink one full recipe of Sassy Water each day.

The ingredients in Sassy Water aren't just for flavor: The ginger helps calm and soothe your GI tract. Even more important, the simple act of making this Sassy Water every day will serve as a reminder during the jumpstart that life is a little bit different and things are going to change.

SASSY WATER

2 liters water (about 8½ cups)
1 teaspoon freshly grated ginger
1 medium cucumber, peeled and thinly sliced
1 medium lemon, thinly sliced
12 small spearmint leaves

Combine all ingredients in a large pitcher and let flavors blend overnight. Drink the entire pitcher by the end of each day.

Eat slowly.

When you eat quickly, you take in large gulps of air, which get trapped in your digestive system and cause bloating.

Avoid the following foods.

The following foods are off-limits for the 4 days of the jumpstart:

- Alcohol, coffee, tea, hot cocoa, and acidic fruit juices
- Bulky raw foods
- Carbonated drinks
- Chewing gum
- Excess carbs
- Fatty foods
- Fried foods
- Gassy foods, including broccoli, Brussels sprouts, cabbage, cauliflower, citrus fruits, legumes, onions, and peppers
- Salt, from the saltshaker, salt-based seasonings, and highly processed foods
- Spicy foods, including foods seasoned with barbecue sauce, black pepper, chile peppers, chili powder, cloves, garlic, horseradish, hot sauce, ketchup, mustard, nutmeg, onions, tomato sauce, or vinegar
- Sugar alcohols, such as xylitol and maltitol, which are often found in low-calorie, low-carb, or sugar-free products such as candy, chewing gum, ice cream, and jam

I CAN'T MAKE A SMOOTHIE AT WORK

The afternoon smoothie presents a challenge for many working men and women. If that's you, I recommend that you pack the ingredients separately, such as 1 cup blueberries, 1 cup fat-free milk, and—instead of the flaxseed oil—2 tablespoons sunflower seeds. Mix them in a bowl or cup. If you choose to do this, get 1 pint fresh instead of frozen blueberries, leave the flaxseed oil off your shopping list, and buy an additional ½ cup sunflower seeds.

YOUR 4-DAY SHOPPING LIST

PRODUCE

- Lemons, 4 medium
- Green beans, 8 ounces fresh or 9 ounces frozen
- Baby carrots, 10-ounce bag
- Cucumbers, 4 medium
- Cremini mushrooms, 2 cups
- Grape tomatoes, 2 pints fresh
- Mint, 2 bunches fresh

DAIRY

- Fat-free milk, ½ gallon
- String cheese, 6-ounce package light or low-fat*

FROZEN FOOD

- Blueberries, 2 (10-ounce) bags frozen unsweetened

DRY GOODS

- Corn flakes, such as Erewhon or Nature's Path, 12-ounce box unsweetened
- Flaxseed oil, 8-ounce bottle cold-pressed organic
- Extra virgin olive oil, 8-ounce bottle
- Sunflower seeds, without the shell, 1 cup bulk or 9-ounce package roasted or raw unsalted
- Applesauce, 4 (4-ounce) cups or 16-ounce jar unsweetened
- Pineapple tidbits packed in juice, 2 (4-ounce) cups or 8-ounce can
- Raisins, 6 (1-ounce) boxes or ¼ cup bulk unsweetened
- Instant Cream of Wheat, 12-ounce box
- Cooking spray, 7.2-ounce can
- Brown rice, 14-ounce box

SPICES

- Ginger, 1–2 knuckles fresh

MEAT/SEAFOOD

- Chicken breast, 9 ounces uncooked boneless, skinless
- Organic deli roast turkey, 8-ounce package low-sodium**
- Tilapia or other mild white fish, 11 ounces uncooked
- Chunk light tuna in water, 6-ounce can or 2 (3-ounce) cans

ANY OF THESE APPROVED SALT-FREE SEASONINGS

If you want to add flavor to your food, use some of these *Flat Belly Diet*–approved salt-free seasonings and herbs with your meals:

- Original and Italian medley Mrs. Dash salt-free seasoning blends
- Fresh or dried: basil, bay leaf, cinnamon, curry powder, dill, ginger, lemon or lime juice, marjoram, mint, oregano, paprika, rosemary, sage, tarragon, or thyme

*We call for light or low-fat string cheese rather than part-skim because it is lower in saturated fat and calories. If you have trouble finding light or low-fat string cheese, though, feel free to substitute with part-skim string cheese.

**Organic deli meat is generally lower in sodium and fat. If your only option is to purchase nonorganic meat, look for low-sodium choices.

SUBSTITUTIONS ON THE JUMPSTART

Because the 4-day jumpstart targets belly bloat and water retention, it is the most limited portion of the *Flat Belly Diet*. We encourage you to follow the meal plan exactly, but if you are allergic to one of these foods or have special dietary needs, use one of these jumpstart-approved substitutes instead. Note that all of the foods in each row are interchangeable with each other. Simply match the exact amounts mentioned here and swap away.

JUMPSTART MENU ITEM	JUMPSTART-APPROVED SUBSTITUTE
PRODUCE	
Grape tomatoes, 1 pint fresh Green beans, 1 cup steamed Cremini mushrooms, 1 cup sautéed Baby carrots, 1 cup steamed	Yellow squash, 1 cup, sautéed
DAIRY	
Fat-free milk, 1 cup	Soy milk, such as Soy Dream (dairy-free, vegan), 1 cup plain unsweetened
	Rice milk, such as Rice Dream (dairy-free, vegan), 1 cup plain enriched
	Almond milk, such as Almond Breeze (vegan), 1 cup
	Lactaid fat-free milk (lactose-free), 1 cup
	Trader Joe's Rice Drink (dairy-free, vegan), 1 cup
String cheese, 1 light or low-fat	Tofutti Veggie Slices, 1 oz
	Galaxy Nutritional Foods Vegan Slices (dairy-free, vegan), 1 oz
FROZEN FOOD	
Blueberries, 1 cup frozen unsweetened Pineapple tidbits packed in juice, 4 oz	Strawberries, 1 cup frozen unsweetened Peaches, 1 cup frozen unsweetened

JUMPSTART MENU ITEM	JUMPSTART-APPROVED SUBSTITUTE
DRY GOODS	
Corn flakes, 1 cup unsweetened Instant Cream of Wheat, 1 packet	Puffed rice cereal, 1 cup unsweetened Gluten-free puffed rice cereal, such as Arrowhead Mills or Erewhon (gluten-free), 1 cup unsweetened Gluten-free corn flakes, such as Health Valley or Nature's Path (gluten-free), 1 cup unsweetened
Flaxseed oil, 1 Tbsp cold-pressed organic	Canola oil, 1 Tbsp Walnut oil, 1 Tbsp Pumpkin seeds, 1½ Tbsp Sunflower seeds, 2 Tbsp
Sunflower seeds, ¼ cup roasted or raw, without the shell	Pumpkin seeds, ¼ cup unsalted without the shell
Applesauce, ½ cup unsweetened Raisins, 2 Tbsp unsweetened	Pineapple tidbits packed in juice, 4 oz
Brown rice, ½ cup cooked	Red potatoes, ½ cup roasted
MEAT/SEAFOOD	
Organic deli roast turkey, 4 oz low-sodium Chunk light tuna in water, 3 oz Tilapia, 4 oz grilled Chicken breast, 3 oz grilled	Turkey slices, such as Applegate Farms (gluten-free), 4 oz Tofurky deli slices (vegan), 4 oz Amy's Kitchen California Veggie Burger (vegan), 1 Gardenburger GardenVegan Burger (vegan), 1

Note: In your jumpstart dinners, you are allowed only 1 teaspoon olive oil, which you can use in any way you'd like to help cook and flavor your foods; in other words, either you can use it to cook your vegetables or meat, or you can drizzle it over them. For other cooking, use the cooking spray.

THE 4-DAY ANTI-BLOAT JUMPSTART MENU

BREAKFAST

1 cup unsweetened corn flakes

1 cup fat-free milk

$\frac{1}{4}$ cup roasted or raw unsalted sunflower seeds

4 ounces ($\frac{1}{2}$ cup) unsweetened applesauce

Glass of Sassy Water

LUNCH

4 ounces deli turkey

1 pint fresh grape tomatoes

1 low-fat string cheese

Glass of Sassy Water

SNACK

Blueberry Smoothie: Blend 1 cup fat-free milk and 1 cup frozen unsweetened blueberries in a blender for 1 minute. Transfer to a glass and stir in 1 tablespoon cold-pressed organic flaxseed oil or serve with 2 tablespoons sunflower seeds, without the shell.

DINNER

4 ounces grilled tilapia, drizzled with 1 teaspoon olive oil

1 cup steamed green beans

$\frac{1}{2}$ cup cooked brown rice

Glass of Sassy Water

THE 4-DAY
ANTI-BLOAT JUMPSTART MENU

BREAKFAST

1 packet instant Cream of Wheat

1 cup fat-free milk

$\frac{1}{4}$ cup roasted or raw unsalted sunflower seeds

2 tablespoons unsweetened raisins

Glass of Sassy Water

LUNCH

3 ounces chunk light tuna in water, drained

1 cup steamed baby carrots

1 low-fat string cheese

Glass of Sassy Water

SNACK

Pineapple Smoothie: Blend 1 cup fat-free milk, 4 ounces canned pineapple tidbits in juice, and a handful of ice in a blender for 1 minute. Transfer to a glass and stir in 1 tablespoon cold-pressed organic flaxseed oil or serve with 2 tablespoons sunflower seeds, without the shell.

DINNER

3 ounces grilled chicken breast, drizzled with 1 teaspoon olive oil

1 cup cremini mushrooms, sautéed in cooking spray, if desired

$\frac{1}{2}$ cup cooked brown rice

Glass of Sassy Water

THE 4-DAY
ANTI-BLOAT JUMPSTART MENU

BREAKFAST

1 cup unsweetened corn flakes

1 cup fat-free milk

¼ cup roasted or raw unsalted sunflower seeds

2 tablespoons unsweetened raisins

Glass of Sassy Water

LUNCH

4 ounces deli turkey

1 cup steamed baby carrots

1 low-fat string cheese

Glass of Sassy Water

SNACK

Blueberry Smoothie: Blend 1 cup fat-free milk and 1 cup frozen unsweetened blueberries in a blender for 1 minute. Transfer to a glass and stir in 1 tablespoon cold-pressed organic flaxseed oil or serve with 2 tablespoons sunflower seeds, without the shell.

DINNER

4 ounces grilled tilapia, drizzled with 1 teaspoon olive oil

1 cup cremini mushrooms, sautéed in cooking spray, if desired

½ cup cooked brown rice

Glass of Sassy Water

THE 4-DAY
ANTI-BLOAT JUMPSTART MENU

BREAKFAST

1 packet instant Cream of Wheat

1 cup fat-free milk

1/4 cup roasted or raw unsalted sunflower seeds

4 ounces (1/2 cup) unsweetened applesauce

Glass of Sassy Water

LUNCH

3 ounces chunk light tuna in water, drained

1 pint fresh grape tomatoes

1 low-fat string cheese

Glass of Sassy Water

SNACK

Pineapple Smoothie: Blend 1 cup fat-free milk, 4 ounces canned pineapple tidbits in juice, and a handful of ice in a blender for 1 minute. Transfer to a glass and stir in 1 tablespoon cold-pressed organic flaxseed oil or serve with 2 tablespoons sunflower seeds, without the shell.

DINNER

3 ounces grilled chicken breast, drizzled with 1 teaspoon olive oil

1 cup steamed green beans

1/2 cup cooked brown rice

Glass of Sassy Water

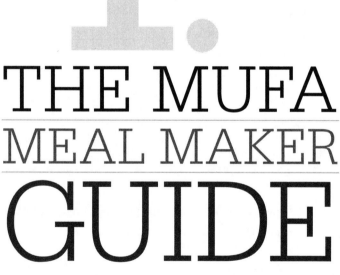

4.

THE MUFA
MEAL MAKER
GUIDE

As we noted in the Introduction, Your Ultimate 28-Day Eating Plan in Chapter 5 is designed to give you a balanced variety of foods with plenty of MUFA-rich foods to flatten your belly, ward off disease, and keep you satisfied and healthy. But you probably don't want to eat the same meals for the rest of your life! Not to worry. The choices for MUFA-packed, delicious meals are limitless. In this section, we give you the guidelines we followed in creating the *Flat Belly Diet* meals so that you can create your own if you choose, using all your favorite foods and fat-blasting MUFAs such as oils, nuts and seeds, avocados, olives, and dark chocolate.

THE BUILDING BLOCKS OF A *FLAT BELLY DIET* MEAL

As you might recall from Chapter 2: The *Flat Belly Diet* at a Glance, there are three simple rules you need to keep in mind on the diet:

Rule #1: Stick to 400 calories per meal.

Rule #2: Never go more than 4 hours without eating.

Rule #3: Eat a MUFA at every meal.

So, what else can you eat with those delicious MUFAs? The beauty of the *Flat Belly Diet* is that almost nothing is forbidden, so you can eat all your favorite foods and be as creative as you like in putting together your meals. But in order to get the most benefit from your MUFA-rich foods, it helps to pair them with lean proteins, low-fat dairy, fruits and vegetables, starches, and whole grains—which just happen to be the basis for a healthy Mediterranean-style diet.

Flat Belly Diet meals are balanced, with around 35 percent of the calories coming from MUFA-rich fats, 45 percent from carbohydrates, and 20 percent from proteins. But don't let the percentages scare you; creating your own *Flat Belly* meals is easy—no math required! You start by selecting your MUFA, and then you simply "build" your meal by adding lean proteins, whole grains or fruit, and (for lunch or dinner) vegetables. Refer to Your MUFA Serving Chart on page 132 for the full list of MUFAs you can choose from.

Here's how to build a *Flat Belly Diet* meal. Visual cues are provided in parentheses.

If your chosen MUFA is oil, nuts, or seeds, pair it with:

- 3 ounces lean protein (about the size of a deck of cards)
- ½ cup cooked whole grain, such as brown or wild rice (mini fruit cup size), *or* 1 whole grain bread serving, such as half of a whole wheat pita, *or* 1 cup fruit (1 baseball)
- 2 cups raw or steamed veggies (2 baseballs)

Example: 3 ounces grilled salmon served over ½ cup whole wheat couscous mixed with 2 tablespoons toasted pine nuts. Serve with 2 cups steamed mixed vegetables.

If your chosen MUFA is avocado or olives, pair it with:

- 3 ounces lean protein (deck of cards) *or* 2 ounces lean protein and 1 dairy, such as 1 slice cheese or ¼ cup shredded or crumbled cheese
- 2 cups raw or steamed veggies (2 baseballs)
- 1 cup starchy vegetables, such as beans, corn, peas, or potatoes, *or* ½ cup cooked whole grain *or* 1 whole grain bread serving, such as half of a whole wheat pita or wrap or 1 slice whole grain bread

Example: 1 slice toasted whole grain bread topped with ¼ cup sliced avocado and 3 ounces roasted chicken. Serve with 2 cups steamed broccoli with a spritz of fresh lemon.

If your chosen MUFA is dark chocolate, such as ¼ cup semisweet or dark chocolate chips, pair it with:

- 1 cup fruit
- 1 cup dairy, such as fat-free cottage cheese or fat-free plain yogurt, *or* 6 ounces fat-free flavored yogurt *or* 1 cup whole grain, such as oatmeal, *or* 2 whole grain waffles

Example: Melt ¼ cup semisweet or dark chocolate chips and drizzle over 1 cup sliced strawberries. Serve with 1 cup fat-free plain yogurt.

In addition to Your MUFA Serving Chart on page 132, you'll find two quick reference lists at the end of the book—Eat These Foods Regularly on page 134 and Eat These Foods Sparingly on page 144—with appropriate serving sizes and calorie counts for all of your meal

FOOD LABEL KNOW-HOW

The Nutrition Facts labels on packaged foods can help you make *Flat Belly Diet*-friendly choices in the grocery store. Here's what to keep your eye on:

Serving Size: It's important to make the serving size one of the first things you check on the label so that you know exactly what's in the package; use the "Servings Per Container" to double-check the amount. So if you have a container of ice cream listing "Servings Per Container: 4," and you plan to eat the entire container, you should multiply the calories (and everything else) by four.

Saturated Fat: The *Flat Belly Diet* saturated fat limit is no more than 3 to 4 grams per 400-calorie meal. Saturated fat content can vary considerably from brand to brand, so read labels and always select packaged products with little or no saturated fat listed on the label.

Trans Fat: Trans fat should be avoided on the *Flat Belly Diet*.

Look for products with 0 grams of trans fat listed on the label. Also check the ingredients list for the trans fat key words *hydrogenated, partially hydrogenated,* and *shortening.* Manufacturers are allowed to claim 0 trans fat for any food actually containing up to $\frac{1}{2}$ gram per serving, so it's important to identify trans fats in the ingredients list.

Sodium: The *Flat Belly Diet* works best when you keep your total sodium below 2,300 milligrams a day. Because sodium content can vary considerably from brand to brand, it's important to read labels and to always select the lower-sodium product.

MUFA-Rich Ingredients: Since MUFAs usually aren't listed on the food label, the best way to spot them in packaged foods is to look at the ingredients lists. Look for MUFA-packed foods like oils, nuts, legumes (edamame and peanuts) and seeds, avocados, olives, and dark chocolate.

building blocks so that it's easy for you to calculate the amount of food you need for each meal.

Note: Foods that include a MUFA in the ingredients are not considered a MUFA for the purposes of building a *Flat Belly Diet* meal. Stick with the MUFAs (and their respective serving sizes) in Your MUFA Serving Chart on page 132 for the MUFA component of your meal.

We also give you a chart of Common Conversions on page 131 to make it easy to measure your servings and help you stay within your 400-calorie limit per meal.

HOW TO SHOP FOR, STORE, AND USE MUFAS

The more you know about your MUFAs, the easier it is to make the *Flat Belly Diet* work for you! To get the most MUFA for your money, use the following tips and tricks for shopping, storing, and using MUFA-rich foods, including oils, nuts, seeds, avocados, olives, and our favorite MUFA: dark chocolate.

MEASURING YOUR MUFAS

Dieters who guesstimate the amounts they eat of calorie-dense MUFA-rich foods are making a big *Flat Belly Diet* no-no, since overestimating can seriously delay progress. For example, if you drizzle 2 tablespoons of olive oil over your salad (instead of the proper 1-tablespoon MUFA allowance), you'll get around 120 extra calories. Yikes. Research shows that most people underestimate serving sizes when eyeballing them, so get in the habit of measuring not only your MUFAs but all of your *Flat Belly Diet* food. It's easy enough to stash a tablespoon in your purse or briefcase so that you can do this when you're out and about. This will help you control not only your portions but also your hunger, to give you the health and weight loss results you're after.

MUFA #1: Oils

Plant-based oils are an important part of your *Flat Belly Diet*. Low in saturated fat and packed with good-for-you MUFAs, they're a delicious way to up your MUFA intake.

Shopping and Storing: Because all MUFA-rich oils are sensitive to heat, light, and air and will go rancid if exposed to these elements or kept too long, it's important to buy in small amounts (only what you will use within a couple of months) and store properly. Select expeller-pressed or cold-pressed oils whenever possible, and store them in a cool, dark place in the back of your pantry or in the refrigerator. Although some, like olive oil, will thicken when chilled, this does no harm to the oils, and they will resume liquid form when they return to room temperature.

Using: From robust and hearty to fragile and delicate, MUFA oils can be included in your diet in a variety of tasty ways.

- **Olive oil.** Drizzle extra virgin olive oil on salads, veggies, and finished dishes, including pasta and grilled meats and fish. It's made from higher-quality, more freshly picked olives through a process that does not involve chemicals, so its fruity flavor and beneficial nutrients are uncompromised. Try using less expensive olive oils for cooking with moderate heat (sautéing or roasting below 375°F; medium on the stovetop).

- **Canola oil.** Versatile and neutral flavored, canola oil is perfect for cooking that requires moderately high heat (up to about 435°F), including baking.

- **Refined peanut oil.** With a high heat tolerance (up to about 450°F) and neutral flavor, this oil is ideal for sautéing or roasting at high temperatures and grilling over direct heat.

- **Sesame oil.** This strongly flavored oil adds an intense taste to marinades, dipping sauces, dressings, and stir-fries.

- **High-oleic safflower and sunflower oils.** Look for natural, unrefined safflower and sunflower oils that specify "high-oleic" on the

A MUFA MUST: PESTO

Pesto—a sauce made with olive oil, herbs, garlic, Parmesan, and pine nuts—is a MUFA must-have. You can make your own (see recipe on page 122 in the *Flat Belly Diet! Cookbook*), or you can buy it already prepared, like Classico Sun-Dried Tomato Pesto or Buitoni Pesto with Basil. Keep in mind that pesto is packed not only with flavor but also with calories (around 50 to 80 calories per tablespoon), and a little goes a long way. Mix a tablespoon or two with pasta, spread some on a sandwich, or spoon it over grilled fish or chicken for a MUFA-dense delicious meal.

label. This means the oils are made from plants bred to have much higher MUFA concentrations than regular safflower and sunflower oils. These mild-tasting oils won't congeal when chilled, making them ideal for dressing cold dishes like pasta salads.

○ **Walnut oil.** Strongly flavored and heat resistant, this pricey oil is best used as a flavoring agent for special dishes.

○ **Flaxseed oil.** Fragile and nutty-flavored flaxseed oil has stellar nutritional benefits, but those properties are lost when the oil is heated, so it is not suited for cooking. Select cold-pressed oil, keep it refrigerated, and try swirling it into a cold soup or vegetable dip, adding it to smoothies, or drizzling over a salad of delicate greens.

MUFA #2: Nuts and Seeds

Packed with protein, flavor, and (of course!) MUFAs, nuts, legumes, and seeds are practical and portable sources of MUFAs.

NUTS

Shopping and Storing

UNSHELLED: Buying nuts whole, with their natural protective covering intact, not only ensures freshness but is also much more economical than buying shelled nuts. Whole nuts can be stored in a cool, dark place for 2 to 3 months.

SHELLED: Shelled nuts (no cracking required) are sold in the baking and snack aisles of the supermarket, as well as in natural and specialty organic food stores, where you'll find a larger variety and better quality of nuts. Select unsalted nuts, raw or roasted without oil. Store them in airtight containers in the refrigerator for up to 3 to 4 months or well wrapped in the freezer for up to a year.

Using: Convenient and portable, nuts are a perfect on-the-go MUFA. Toss them into your purse, suitcase, or gym bag for an anytime snack or meal addition. As you'll see in Your MUFA Serving Chart (on page 132), the serving size for most nuts is 2 tablespoons; you may want to measure that amount into small zip-top plastic bags—or simply carry a tablespoon with you. Nuts are a crunchy and MUFA-rich way to jazz up just about any dish.

- **Almonds.** Whether dry roasted, raw, sliced, blanched, slivered, or chopped, this versatile nut can be tossed into vegetable salads, granolas and mueslis, fruit salads, and grain-based salads. Almonds can also be used in baking, ground to top or encrust fish fillets or chicken breasts, or pureed with herbs for a pesto alternative.

- **Brazil nuts.** These large tree nuts have a mild flavor and rich, coconut-like texture, and they can be coarsely chopped and mixed with rice pilaf or grain-based salads (such as quinoa, bulgur, or brown rice).

- **Cashews.** With a deep flavor and creamy texture, these nuts are perfectly paired with fruit, salads, stir-fries, and curried dishes.

- **Hazelnuts (filberts).** Their sweet flavor makes them especially suited for baked goods and sweet dishes. Also try them added to granolas and mueslis, fruit salads, pilafs, grain-based salads, and spinach salads.

- **Macadamia nuts.** These buttery, decadent-tasting nuts pair brilliantly with tropical fruits like pineapple, kiwifruit, and mango and with mild-flavored fish, including halibut, sole, tilapia, cod, and mahi mahi.

- **Pecans.** With a rich, sweet flavor and a classic crunch, these nuts are a natural not only with desserts but also with spinach salads, rich pureed soups, roasted squash, baked apples, and crisp-tender vegetables. Also try them stirred into waffle, pancake, or muffin batter.

- **Pine nuts.** These nutlike seeds are best pureed in pesto, toasted and tossed into salads and pasta dishes, stirred into grain dishes, or mixed with sautéed greens like spinach, kale, or chard.

- **Pistachios.** These crunchy nuts are delicious mixed in savory dishes like pasta, chicken salads, and grain dishes.

TOASTY AND TASTY

Toasting nuts releases their natural oils, which not only enhances the aroma and flavor but also makes their texture crunchier. Toasting nuts at home is easier than you think. Here's how.

In the oven: Preheat the oven to 250°F. Spread shelled nuts on a baking sheet and bake for 1 to 2 minutes. Shake the pan and continue to bake for 1 to 2 minutes longer or until the nuts start to turn light brown. Immediately remove from the oven.

On the stovetop: Place shelled nuts in a heavy skillet on the stovetop. Heat the skillet slowly over medium heat (shaking the pan continuously), until the nuts start to turn light brown—2 to 4 minutes. Remove from the heat immediately.

Keep in mind that toasting nuts is a process that starts slowly, but ends quickly. Burning makes nuts taste bitter, so be sure to remove them from the heat as soon as they start to turn color. They will continue to cook as they cool.

A MUFA MUST: NUT BUTTERS

Tried-and-true peanut butter is a MUFA-packed superstar, but to mix things up, why not try nut butters like almond and cashew? No matter what nut butter you use, be sure to buy all-natural brands in order to avoid emulsifiers and other unhealthy additives. Look for nut butters whose ingredients list shows just nuts and maybe a little salt, oil, or a touch of sugar or honey, such as Futters Nut Butters.

○ **Walnuts.** With a longer shelf life (9 to 12 months in the refrigerator) than many other nuts, they make a good staple nut to stock in the kitchen. Use them crumbled onto salads, pasta, and soups; pureed into a hummuslike dip; or tossed with rolled oats.

LEGUMES

Not all legumes (plants that bear fruit in the form of a pod that opens along two seams) are good sources of MUFAs. Some, such as beans, peas, and lentils, are fantastic sources of protein and other nutrients, so you should definitely include them in your diet, but they don't contain MUFAs. Edamame (green soybeans) and peanuts, however, are MUFA-packed exceptions.

EDAMAME

Shopping and Storing: While fresh soybeans (deep green fuzzy pods) are sometimes available at local farmers' markets, frozen edamame are almost always available at large supermarkets. You can get them shelled and cooked, whole and cooked, or whole and uncooked.

Using

UNSHELLED: The outside pods aren't edible, but eating your edamame straight from pod to mouth is a fun (and authentically Japanese) way to enjoy these legumes. Just hold the pod lengthwise near your lips and pinch its outer edge to press the beans against the inner seam, which will split so the beans pop into your mouth. Two cups unshelled edamame is equivalent to 1 cup shelled (which is 1 MUFA serving).

SHELLED: Shelled and cooked soybeans are a perfect complement to whole grains, meats, salads, soups, and vegetable dishes. They team up especially well with Asian-inspired meals.

PEANUTS

Shopping and Storing: You can choose from whole or shelled; skin-on or blanched; raw, dry roasted, or boiled. Like tree nuts, whole unshelled peanuts can be stored in a cool, dark place for 2 to 3 months, and shelled peanuts can be stored in airtight containers in the refrigerator for up to 3 to 4 months or wrapped in the freezer for up to a year.

Using: Whether whole, halved, chopped, roasted, or raw, peanuts can be included in stir-fries, salads, whole grain dishes, and whole wheat noodle salads. They can also be used in dressings, dips, and baked goods.

SEEDS

Shopping and Storing: As with nuts, you will find a larger and fresher selection of seeds in natural and specialty organic food stores. Whole seeds should be kept in airtight containers in the refrigerator and taste best if they are consumed within a couple of months. Once ground, seeds go bad very quickly, sometimes within a few days.

A MUFA MUST: TAHINI

Tahini, a Middle Eastern pantry staple, is a creamy paste made from ground sesame seeds. It's available roasted or plain in the ethnic food section of most supermarkets. It's also an ingredient in spreads and hummus (any flavor), such as Sabra Tahini Spread and Dip. Try it as a dip for veggies, a spread for sandwiches, and a dressing for salads when mixed with oil, vinegar or lemon juice, parsley, and garlic.

A MUFA MUST: GUACAMOLE

Guacamole is a dip made with ripe avocados mashed with tomatoes, onion, cilantro, jalapeño chile peppers, and lime juice. You can whip up your own (see recipe on page 59) or look for supermarket brands like AvoClassic and Wholly Guacamole that list real avocados as the first ingredient. Use it as a dip, in burritos, or as an interesting sandwich topping.

Using: Snack on them out of hand or use whole toasted seeds sprinkled on cereal, yogurt, and fruit; tossed into green salads; stirred into tuna, chicken, or turkey salad; or added to savory baked goods. Raw kernels can be sprinkled over breads and muffins before baking and sautéed with vegetables, and ground seeds can be folded into veggie or turkey burger mix or used as a base for sauces and dips.

MUFA #3: Avocados

This super-creamy fruit is not only packed with MUFAs but is also high in cancer-fighting carotenoids. It's a decidedly decadent and healthy way to get a MUFA in every meal.

Shopping and Storing: Avocados are typically available in two varieties—the Hass or California (pebbled green skin that turns dark brown as the fruit ripens) and the larger Florida variety (smooth green skin). For either variety, buying unripe or just barely ripe ensures the best flavor and texture: Pick fruits that are quite firm or give only ever so slightly to a gentle squeeze. Ripening at room temperature usually takes just a day or two (no more than three or four at most), and putting the fruit in a brown bag can speed the ripening process by about a day. Once ripe, refrigerate and use within a day or two.

Using: Spread it like butter on bread, sandwiches, and burgers; mash it into dips; and use it sliced or chopped in salads and wraps.

Avocados pair particularly well with Mexican-themed dishes like quesadillas, taco salads, and fajitas.

MUFA #4: Olives

These Mediterranean gems are not only chock-full of MUFAs but also rich in vitamin E, an antioxidant that protects cell membranes and reduces inflammation. From green, black, or brown to Spanish, Greek, and California, there are plenty of ways to incorporate olives into your life.

Shopping and Storing: Olives are found all over the supermarket—look for them in the condiment/pickle aisle, the natural foods section, the deli, and the international department. For the best flavor and texture, whenever possible select unpasteurized fresh olives over pasteurized jarred varieties and choose whole olives over pitted. They can be kept in airtight containers at room temperature, but they'll last longer when stored in the refrigerator.

Using: Whole, pitted, or sliced olives are a wonderful snack and a tangy addition to salads, stewed chicken and meat dishes, and pasta sauces.

MUFA #5: Dark Chocolate

A diet that encourages you to eat chocolate? You bet! Dark chocolate is a rich source of MUFAs and, if consumed in (ahem) reasonable

A MUFA MUST: TAPENADE

Traditional tapenade is a delightful mix of chopped olives, olive oil, and seasonings. Used as a spread, sauce, or condiment, it's easy to prepare your own (see recipe on page 181 of the *Flat Belly Diet! Cookbook*) and even easier to pick up packaged tapenade in the supermarket. Beware of artichoke, eggplant, and other tapenade impostors; instead opt for olive tapenades, like Mt. Vikos Kalamata Olive Spread or Cantaré Olive Tapenade, that list olives as the main ingredient and have around 40 calories per tablespoon.

quantities, a healthy and enjoyable component of the *Flat Belly Diet.*

Shopping and Storing: You can buy your dark chocolate in chunks, bars, or chips. Look for chocolate with at least 60 percent cacao, and keep in mind that heat affects flavor and consistency, so your favorite eating chocolate may not be the best performer as a baking chocolate. Chocolate should be stored in its original wrapping in a cool, dry place (but not in the fridge, which is too cold and moist) and away from strong-smelling items (chocolate absorbs odors). Stored properly, most dark chocolate will last up to a year.

Using: Dark chocolate is divine all on its own, of course, but it can also be swirled into oatmeal; mixed into muffin, waffle, and pancake batter; sprinkled into yogurt; and eaten with fruit.

WHAT ELSE CAN I EAT?

In addition to a delicious "MUFA at every meal," your *Flat Belly Diet* is packed with lots of other hearty and wholesome foods that will keep you feeling satisfied and hunger free. As we noted earlier, there are no forbidden foods on the *Flat Belly Diet,* but you do want your meals to be a balanced mix of MUFA-rich fats; good-for-you carbohydrates, including whole grains, fruits, and vegetables; and lean proteins, like fish, chicken, beans, and low-fat dairy. This combination of foods, eaten at regular intervals (every 4 hours), will keep you burning belly fat, while maintaining energy, muscle mass, and bone density.

Here are a few general guidelines to keep in mind to help you eat and lose weight the *Flat Belly Diet* way.

Guideline #1: Consume no more than 4 grams of saturated fat per meal.

Saturated fat raises levels of LDL ("bad" cholesterol) in your blood and, in turn, increases your risk of cardiovascular disease and stroke. Animal products, like meat and dairy products, are the main sources of saturated fat, but tropical oils—coconut oil and palm (or palm kernel) oil—and cocoa butter are also high in saturated fat. Small amounts of saturated fat are also found in some other plant foods, including MUFA-rich olive oil and nuts, so it's impossible to eliminate the saturated fats altogether. However, you can greatly decrease the amount in your diet by

THE "FAT" FACTS OF DARK CHOCOLATE

With the limit on saturated fats, you might be wondering why dark chocolate is included in the *Flat Belly Diet* plan, since the amount we recommend (¼ cup of chocolate chips or the equivalent) contains quite a bit more than 3 grams of saturated fat. There are different types of saturated fat, and the type in dark chocolate (stearic acid) largely gets converted in the body to oleic acid, which is a MUFA! So although dark chocolate has a higher saturated fat content—and when you include it in one of your *Flat Belly Diet* meals, your total saturated fat will be over the 4-gram max— this type does not tend to raise blood cholesterol levels and is considered heart healthy.

substituting healthier fats, like olive oil and canola oil, for straight saturated fats like butter. In Your Ultimate 28-Day Eating Plan, we've kept the saturated fat level as low as possible (around 3 grams per meal), so you see it *is* possible to have flavor without saturated fats!

Guideline #2: Ban trans fat.

Like saturated fat, trans fat increases levels of LDL ("bad" cholesterol) in your blood. But that's not all. Trans fat also lowers levels of HDL ("good" cholesterol), which helps keep blood vessels clear, making trans fat a really bad fat. Trans fat is produced when hydrogen is added to liquid oils to make them solid (and extend their shelf life), and it is found mostly in packaged products. Because manufacturers are allowed to claim zero trans fat for any food actually containing up to half a gram per serving, it's important to identify trans fats in the ingredients list. Look for the words *hydrogenated, partially hydrogenated,* and *shortening.* If you spot these terms in the list, put that food down and keep looking!

Guideline #3: Avoid artificial sweeteners, flavorings, and preservatives.

Aspartame is one of the most prevalent artificial sweeteners used in foods and drinks today. It's found in diet sodas, sugar-free yogurts and puddings, chewable vitamins, gum, and even high-fiber cereal. But ever since the FDA approved it in 1981, many nutrition researchers have disputed its safety and many people have complained that it causes headaches, dizziness, and mood changes. Artificial food colorings used in some sugary cereals and candies have been linked to hyperactivity and behavior problems since the 1970s. Nitrates, which add flavor (mostly to meats), have been linked to various types of cancer. And these are just a few of the many artificial additives in our food. Try to avoid artificial anything (colors, flavors, preservatives); instead pick whole foods as often as possible and look for foods with ingredients you can easily recognize and pronounce. The *Flat Belly Diet*–Friendly Products list (page 105) can also help you identify additive-free packaged foods.

Guideline #4: Limit sodium to less than 2,300 milligrams a day.

Sodium causes water retention (which not only makes your weight temporarily spike on the scale but also causes unsightly puffiness) and increases your risk for high blood pressure, which can lead to

BE SAVVY ABOUT SODIUM

Keeping your *Flat Belly Diet* sodium below 2,300 milligrams per day is a snap. Here's how:

○ **Limit salty MUFAs.** While most MUFAs are low in sodium, olives are indisputably salty, so it's best to limit olives (and olive dishes) to no more than once a day. Also read the labels carefully on packaged MUFA-rich foods like olive-based tapenade, pesto, and nut butters, and always pick the lower-sodium products.

○ **Ditch the shaker.** Put away the saltshaker and use the following *Flat Belly Diet*–approved (sodium-free) seasonings instead: fresh or dried basil, dill, ginger, marjoram, mint, oregano, rosemary, sage, tarragon, and thyme as well as aged balsamic vinegar (use lightly: 1 tablespoon = 5 calories), bay leaf, cinnamon, curry powder, lemon or lime juice,

paprika, and salt-free seasoning blends such as Mrs. Dash.

○ **Go whole.** The *Flat Belly Diet* encourages you to limit highly processed foods (they are the main source of excessive sodium in the average American diet) and instead to use real foods made from whole ingredients like fruits, vegetables, whole grains, and lean proteins.

○ **Read labels.** When you do purchase packaged foods (like bread, canned beans, sauces, and MUFA-rich nut butters and tapenade), always compare brands. Sodium content can vary considerably from brand to brand, so read labels and always select the lower-sodium product. And be sure to rinse canned beans, vegetables, and tuna in a colander under cool running water for 2 to 3 minutes to remove up to 30 percent of the sodium.

heart and kidney disease, as well as stroke. Because the *Flat Belly Diet* is about flattening your belly *and* enhancing good health, the *Flat Belly Diet* recommends keeping your total sodium below 2,300 milligrams a day (or approximately 575 milligrams per meal).

HOW TO SHOP FOR, STORE, AND USE THE OTHER MEAL BUILDING BLOCKS

The *Flat Belly Diet* is packed with a variety of delicious and good-for-you foods that, when combined with MUFAs, offer a healthy way to unload belly fat. And the more you know about these nourishing food picks, the more likely you are to embrace this healthful way of eating for a lifetime. To help you get the most out of your *Flat Belly Diet*, use the following tips and tricks for shopping, storing, and using the other *Flat Belly Diet*-friendly foods, including lean proteins, dairy, fruits and vegetables, and whole grains.

Proteins

For good health and weight loss and to keep the saturated fat in your meals within the *Flat Belly* limit of 3 to 4 grams, it's important to always make your protein picks *lean* picks.

BEEF, POULTRY, AND PORK

Shopping and Storing: While beef, poultry, and pork are packed with lots of high-quality protein, if your picks aren't "lean," they can also pack your arteries with a hefty dose of saturated fat. Here's what to look for in the store.

- **Beef:** Pick the leanest cuts, including round steaks and roasts (round eye, top round, bottom round, round tip), tenderloin, sirloin, and chuck shoulder.

- **Poultry:** Pick skinless chicken or turkey parts. Boneless, skinless turkey cutlets and chicken breasts are the leanest picks.

- **Pork:** Select the leanest cuts, including pork loin, tenderloin, center loin, and ham.

- **Ground meat:** Select 90 percent or higher "lean" ground beef and low-fat ground turkey breast or chicken.

- **Cold cuts:** Select lean turkey, chicken, turkey ham, turkey pastrami, or ham. Uncured or preservative-free versions are your best picks.

- **Vegetarian meat substitutes:** Look for veggie burgers, crumbles, etc., with no more than 2 grams of saturated fat (no trans fat) and 480 milligrams of sodium per serving.

Keep in mind that Nutrition Facts labels on fresh meat and poultry are not mandatory, so for even more help making your best picks, simply ask your butcher for nutrition information (most stores carry in-store Nutrition Facts). The color of fresh meat is highly unstable and therefore is not the best indicator of freshness. Instead, pay attention to the smell (fresh, not sour) and the feel (firm, not mushy) of the meat. Also, check use-by and sell-by dates and buy the product with the latest date.

SHOULD I BUY ORGANIC MEAT?

Organic poultry and meat are good choices if you are concerned about antibiotic use and pesticides. Organic meat (marked "USDA Organic" with a round green and white circle) doesn't contain residual pesticides, because the animals must be given pesticide-free organic feed or must graze on land on which pesticides haven't been used for at least 3 years. The animals also can't be given antibiotics nor can they be fed animal by-products. Also, organic meat tends to be lower in sodium and fat. Plus, packaged organic deli meat often lasts longer. For this reason, you'll see that Your Ultimate 28-Day Eating Plan calls for organic meats. If you choose to purchase non-organic meat, please look for low-sodium choices.

Fresh cuts of beef, poultry, and pork can be stored in the refrigerator for 2 to 3 days after the sell-by date and in the freezer for 6 to 12 months. Ground meat can be stored in the freezer only up to 3 months. Try freezing individual pieces of meat or burger patties. They thaw more quickly, and you can pull out one or more depending on your needs, making preparation a snap.

Using: You can roast, braise, broil, grill, or bake your lean cut of meat and use it in a variety of healthy and tasty ways. Use it in a sandwich, toss it into a salad, pair it with pasta, mix it in grain dishes, or serve it all on its own. You can also check out the plethora of delicious MUFA-rich, lean meat recipes featured in the *Flat Belly Diet! Cookbook*.

FISH

Shopping and Storing: Fish is a *Flat Belly Diet* protein-superstar. Loaded with heart-healthy omega-3 fats, it's a high-quality protein source that is low in saturated fat and full of healthful nutrients. Here are a few things to keep in mind.

- ○ When selecting seafood, fatty dark fish (such as salmon, tuna, and bluefish) provide a good source of the omega-3 fats. Light-colored fish (such as orange roughy, snapper, and sole) as well as a variety of shellfish are good choices, too. They're low in fat but high in protein.

- ○ If possible, pick wild fish over farmed fish (farmed fish have higher levels of contaminants than those caught in the wild), but keep in mind that farmed fish is better than no fish at all.

- ○ Breaded or seasoned frozen fish should have no more than 3 grams of saturated fat (0 grams of trans fat) and 480 milligrams of sodium per 4-ounce fillet or serving or 3-ounce cake or burger.

- ○ Buy fish canned in water (not oil), and the lower the sodium, the better. You can also get tuna or salmon in a convenient (no draining needed) vacuum-packed pouch.

When buying whole fish, look for moist skin; bright red, moist gills; firm flesh that bounces back when touched; and clear eyes. When buying fillets, steaks, or shellfish, look for firm flesh, clear color with even coloring, and a moist appearance. Fresh fish is best used within a day or two of purchase and can be frozen for 2 to 3 months.

Using: Use a healthy cooking method (baking, broiling, roasting, braising, grilling, or stir-frying) and allow about 10 minutes of cooking time for every inch of thickness. Like beef, poultry, and pork, fish (and shellfish) can be used in an array of ways. You can toss it into a salad, use it in a sandwich, serve it on its own, or use it in your favorite recipes.

EGGS

Shopping and Storing: Egg whites (two medium eggs yield about ¼ cup of egg whites) and egg substitutes are lean-protein, low-calorie *Flat Belly Diet* picks. Naturally free of fat and cholesterol, egg whites and

DO I NEED TO BE CONCERNED ABOUT MERCURY IN FISH?

The FDA and the Environmental Protection Agency advise only a small group (women who may become pregnant, pregnant women, nursing mothers, and young children) to avoid fish with high levels of contaminants—shark, swordfish, king mackerel, or tilefish—and to limit any kind of fish to no more than two meals a week. The government also recommends this same group restrict canned albacore tuna to no more than 6 ounces per week (canned albacore white tuna has three times more mercury than light). While this group is *especially* vulnerable to contamination, all of us are at risk and should follow the government's recommendations accordingly.

THE MUFA MEAL MAKER GUIDE

WHAT IF I'M VEGETARIAN OR VEGAN?

The *Flat Belly Diet* is vegan and vegetarian friendly. We've given you vegan substitutions for the ingredients on the jumpstart plan (page 14). You can also select vegan and vegetarian alternatives, such as beans and lentils, in place of meat and fish in any meal during the 28-day plan. Just be sure to match the calories and keep each meal to about 400 calories. See the list of meat alternatives in the *Flat Belly Diet*-Friendly Products list on page 107.

egg substitutes like Organic Valley, Better'n Eggs, All Whites, and some Egg Beaters, have just 25 to 30 calories per $\frac{1}{4}$ cup.

Using: Use them in an omelet, a frittata, or a quiche; scramble them with veggies, lean meats, or low-fat cheese; fill a burrito, a sandwich, or a wrap. Egg whites and substitutes can be used in just as many ways as whole eggs.

Dairy

Shopping and Storing: Dairy foods, including milk, yogurt, and cheese, are packed with nutrients needed for good health. In fact, research has shown that a diet rich in dairy foods reduces the risk of osteoporosis—a disease that causes bone fractures later in life. But full-fat dairy foods are loaded with calories and artery-clogging saturated fat. What to do? Simply pick low-fat or fat-free dairy products. You'll get all the vitamins and minerals you'd get from whole-milk products but without all of the extra calories and bad-for-you fat. In the store:

- Choose 1% or fat-free milk.

- Select low-fat or fat-free yogurt with no more than 2 grams of saturated fat per $\frac{1}{2}$-cup serving.

- Choose low-fat or fat-free cheese (including hard cheese, string cheese, cream cheese, cheese spreads, and goat cheese) with no more than 2 or 3 grams of saturated fat per 1-ounce serving ($\frac{1}{2}$ cup of cottage cheese or $\frac{1}{4}$ cup of ricotta cheese should have no more than 2 grams of saturated fat).

- Look for low-fat and fat-free versions of other dairy products, including half-and-half, sour cream, and pudding.

When shopping for dairy, always compare prices and brands. Many generic brands offer the same quality as the name brands, but for a lot less money. Also check use-by and sell-by dates and buy the product with the latest date.

Using: While yogurt, cheese, and milk make a perfect anytime snack all on their own, they can also jazz up just about any MUFA-rich meal. Whip up a smoothie with milk, make a parfait with yogurt and fruit, sprinkle grated cheese over your salad or in your soup, or use sliced cheese in a sandwich. The dairy possibilities are endless.

CAN I SUBSTITUTE SOY FOR DAIRY?

Yes, both soy and dairy products (milk, yogurt, cheese, etc.) provide protein, carbohydrates, and nutrients; however, if you pick soy, pick fortified. Calcium-fortified soy "dairy" products have nutrient levels similar to cow's-milk products and are the best substitute for real dairy.

IS ORGANIC PRODUCE BEST?

Eating organic produce does help to reduce your exposure to potentially harmful chemicals, and organic farming is better for the environment. However, if money or availability is an issue, limit your organic produce purchases to the 12 fruits and vegetables the Environmental Working Group deems the most contaminated. The "dirty dozen" are (in order) peaches, apples, bell peppers, celery, nectarines, strawberries, cherries, lettuce, imported grapes, pears, spinach, and potatoes.

Fruits and Vegetables

Shopping and Storing: Naturally delicious and packed with nutrients and filling fiber, fruits and vegetables are an important part of the *Flat Belly Diet*.

○ Choose fresh fruits and vegetables that are firm, unblemished, and in season, when they tend to be less expensive.

○ Use fresh fruits and veggies within a few days after shopping and use frozen or canned produce later in the week.

○ Choose frozen or canned fruits and vegetables without added sugar, fat, or salt.

○ Select whole fruits and vegetables over more expensive precut or prepackaged. When you get home from the store, chop some fresh fruits and vegetables and keep them in the refrigerator so they will be ready to grab for meals and snacks.

○ Buy dried fruits and veggies that are processed without added sugar, fat, or salt.

○ Starchy vegetables like potatoes, beans, lentils, corn, and peas are found not only in the produce aisle but also in the dry food bins, the canned food aisle, and the frozen food section. If you choose frozen or canned starchy vegetables over fresh, be sure to choose no-salt or low-salt varieties and rinse them well before use.

Using: They add crunch, freshness, and flavor to any meal or snack. Raw, roasted, steamed, blanched, or baked, fruits and vegetables can be tossed into salads, used in sandwiches, served as side dishes, made into salsas, and used as desserts. And we're not just talking standard oranges, broccoli, or grapes—these days, supermarkets are packed with a wide assortment of exotic fruits and vegetables, and there's no good reason not to grab a few new varieties on every trip to the store.

Whole Grains

Shopping and Storing: While all grains are good sources of carbohydrates and are naturally low in fat, whole grains—that is, grains that have not had their fiber- and nutrient-rich bran and germ removed by processing—are much, much better. Packed with filling fiber, nutrients, and disease-fighting antioxidants and phytochemicals, whole grain products are always a better bet than refined ones.

Look for bread, cereal, couscous, rice, crackers, pasta, and other grain products that are 100 percent whole grain—meaning they contain *no* refined flours. If the label does not say "100 percent whole grain," flip that package over and investigate the ingredients list.

○ **Whole grain ingredients to look for:** amaranth, barley, brown rice, buckwheat, bulgur wheat, cracked wheat, millet, oats, popcorn, quinoa, rye, spelt, whole wheat, and wild rice

○ **Refined ingredients to avoid:** bleached or unbleached enriched wheat flour, cornmeal, rice flour, semolina or durum flour, white flour, and white rice

Don't be fooled by packages that claim to be an "excellent" or a "good source of" whole grains or by label terms like *seven-grain, multigrain,*

GOOD CARBS, BAD CARBS

The *Flat Belly Diet* is not a *no*-carb or *low*-carb plan. It's a *balanced* plan. Carbohydrates are your body's main energy source and are necessary in the metabolism of essential nutrients. Any diet that eliminates carbohydrates denies the body what it needs to function properly. However, all carbohydrates are not created equal. Your *Flat Belly Diet* is packed with "good" (nutrient-dense) carbohydrates like whole grains, fruits, vegetables, low-fat milk, and beans, instead of "bad" (nutrient-poor) carbs such as refined grains and sugary foods like candy, cookies, soda, and cake.

whole-grain blend, and *made with whole grain.* These foods can contain far more refined grain than whole grain. Always check to see whether the predominant or first ingredient listed is a whole grain.

When deciding on grain products, always compare prices and brands. Like dairy and other packaged products, many generic brands of grains offer the same quality as the name brands, but for a lot less money. Also check use-by and sell-by dates and buy the product with the latest date.

Using: From breakfast (waffles, oatmeal, and toast) to lunch (sandwiches, salads, and soups) to dinner (pilafs, pastas, and side dishes), whole grains can add wholesome flavor to every meal. Check out the *Flat Belly Diet! Cookbook* for lots of fresh ideas.

THE *FLAT BELLY DIET* PANTRY

Now that you have an idea of how to select foods for the *Flat Belly Diet*, here's a summary of a few easy switches to remember the next time you load your shopping cart. Keep these wholesome ingredients on hand in your pantry to make it easy for you to prepare a *Flat Belly Diet* meal any time.

BYPASS	BUY INSTEAD
Corn oil or blended vegetable oil	MUFA-rich oils, such as olive or canola oil
Butter or stick margarine	MUFA-rich spreads such as mashed avocado or hummus
Salted or oil-roasted nuts or seeds	Raw or dry-roasted nuts or seeds without salt
Regular peanut butter	All-natural peanut butter or other nut butter
Milk or white chocolate chips or cocoa powder	Semisweet or dark chocolate chips
85% lean meat	95% lean meat or vegetarian meat substitutes
Whole or 2% milk	Fat-free milk
Whole-milk cheese or yogurt	Light, low-fat, or part-skim cheese or yogurt
Sweetened dried fruit	Unsweetened dried fruit
Canned fruits or vegetables with added sugar, salt, or fat	Canned or frozen fruits or vegetables with no added sugar, salt, or fat
Bleached white flour	Whole wheat or rye flour
Low-fiber cereals and breads	Whole grain cereals and breads with at least 2 to 3 grams of fiber per serving
White, processed pasta	Whole wheat or whole grain pasta
White rice	Brown or wild rice or other whole grains such as barley, millet, oats, or rye
Bottled dressings and marinades	MUFA-rich olive oil and vinegar, such as balsamic or rice vinegar
Bottled sauces or spreads	MUFA-rich sauces or spreads such as pesto, tahini, or olive tapenade

5.

YOUR ULTIMATE
28-DAY
EATING PLAN

In this chapter, you'll find all of the information you've just learned about MUFA-rich foods and other *Flat Belly Diet* meal building blocks wrapped up into a simple and easy-to-follow plan. This plan takes the guesswork out of creating MUFA-rich meals and makes it super-easy to learn how to eat the *Flat Belly Diet* way. Because this plan was created by a registered dietitian, you can be assured that it supplies all of the nutrients you need. Call it the no-brainer *Flat Belly Diet*.

Your Ultimate 28-Day Eating Plan is, of course, based on the three rules of the *Flat Belly Diet*:

Rule #1: Stick to 400 calories per meal.

Rule #2: Never go more than 4 hours without eating.

Rule #3: Eat a MUFA at every meal.

And it's also based on the guidelines we outlined in Chapter 4: The MUFA Meal Maker Guide:

Guideline #1: Consume no more than 4 grams of saturated fat per meal.

Guideline #2: Ban trans fat.

Guideline #3: Avoid artificial sweeteners, flavorings, and preservatives.

Guideline #4: Limit sodium to less than 2,300 milligrams per day.

In this section, you'll find a simple grocery list for each week's worth of meals and a schedule of Quick-and-Easy Meals and Snack Packs, each containing about 400 calories and a MUFA. In each week, you'll see that some of the meals repeat, but trust me, there's enough variety so that you won't get bored. Every week, you'll enjoy three different breakfasts, four lunches, four snacks, and five dinners. What's more, you'll get to try six or seven new MUFAs each week. If you do want a different breakfast, lunch, dinner, and snack every single day, be my guest. There's no rule against it! However, this 28-day meal plan has been specifically designed to maximize your food dollar and prevent wasted leftovers. More variety, of course, means a longer grocery list and more money out of your pocket. So I urge you to give this 28-day plan a try, and if you feel like making a few adjustments, have fun! Chapter 6 contains 30 additional Quick-and-Easy Meals and Snack Packs that can easily be slotted in. Remember, since every meal contains a MUFA and roughly the same number of calories, mixing and matching to create a daily menu you love is easy. And, of course, you can always use recipes from the original *Flat Belly Diet!* book, or create your own based on the guidelines in Chapter 4. One more thing—the 28-day plan has also been designed to save you time; all of the meals can be made in 20 minutes or less and can be made ahead of time. So if you see that Your Ultimate 28-Day Eating Plan calls for Creamy Peanut Soup two times during the week, you can multiply your recipe by two, make one big batch, and eat it throughout the week as indicated.

Now tell me, what could be easier than this?

SWAPPING MADE EASY

Feel like having breakfast for dinner? All of the *Flat Belly Diet* meals and snacks are interchangeable, so you can swap or repeat meals to your heart's content. Bear in mind, though, that it's still important to eat a variety of foods to ensure that you get all the nutrients you need. You can also substitute foods you like within a specific meal for those that you don't. If you prefer to have two slices of whole wheat bread instead of a whole wheat wrap, that's fine! Just match the calories and be sure to choose foods in the same food group to substitute for one another. For example, two slices of bacon are not a substitute for a whole wheat wrap. But $\frac{1}{2}$ cup fresh mango chunks can substitute for 2 tablespoons raisins—they are both fruits and those servings give you about the same number of calories and similar nutritional bang for the buck.

Here's how to substitute.

1. Swap one meal or snack for another. All of the meals and snacks in the 28-day meal plan and the quick meals and snacks are interchangeable because they have all been designed to stay within the 400-calorie-per-meal range, and they are all nutritionally balanced according to the guidelines in the MUFA Meal Maker Guide.

2. Swap one ingredient for another, but select the same category of food. Substitute a vegetable for a vegetable, a whole grain for a whole

ALL-MUFA MEAL

It's tempting to have an all-MUFA meal or snack. But 400 calories of peanut butter right off the spoon or 400 calories of pecans, and so on, well, that's not how this plan works. First, because MUFAs are high in calories, you won't get enough energy from 400 calories' worth of peanut butter to last you the 4 hours until your next meal. Plus, as much as you might enjoy your MUFA-rich foods, they must be combined with the other foods on your meal plan for you to get enough nutrition from the *Flat Belly Diet*. Plus, pairing your MUFAs with other foods helps slow digestion so you feel fuller longer.

grain, a fruit for a fruit, a MUFA for a MUFA, a dairy for a dairy, a lean protein for a lean protein, or a spice/seasoning for a spice/seasoning. The calories are listed in your meal plan in parentheses after the food, so just match the calories and swap the foods. You'll also find three quick reference lists in the back of the book—Your MUFA Serving Chart, Eat These Foods Regularly, and Eat These Foods Sparingly—that list serving sizes and calorie counts so that you can easily find a substitute in your category.

MUFA Swaps

If you don't like or can't find a MUFA, don't despair. Trade these like-calorie MUFAs for one another. Look for the MUFA listed in your meal plan and check out the alternatives below to see if a swap makes sense. I've included only a selection of the most common MUFAs with similar calories, so not all MUFAs are listed here. You will find the complete list of MUFAs in Your MUFA Serving Chart on page 132. Go ahead, swap away!

MUFA CALORIES	MUFA SWAPS
About 50	Green olive tapenade, 2 tablespoons Green or black olives, 10 large
About 80	Pesto sauce, 1 tablespoon Walnuts, 2 tablespoons Florida avocado, ¼ cup
About 90	Pecans, 2 tablespoons Pistachios, 2 tablespoons Sunflower seeds, 2 tablespoons Black olive tapenade, 2 tablespoons
About 100	Cashews, 2 tablespoons Hass avocado, ¼ cup
About 110	Almonds, 2 tablespoons Brazil nuts, 2 tablespoons Hazelnuts, 2 tablespoons Pine nuts, 2 tablespoons Peanuts, 2 tablespoons
About 120	Canola oil, 1 tablespoon Flaxseed oil (cold-pressed organic), 1 tablespoon Olive oil, 1 tablespoon Peanut oil, 1 tablespoon Safflower oil (high oleic), 1 tablespoon Sesame or soybean oil, 1 tablespoon Sunflower oil (high oleic), 1 tablespoon Walnut oil, 1 tablespoon Macadamia nuts, 2 tablespoons
About 190	Cashew butter, 2 tablespoons Sunflower seed butter, 2 tablespoons Peanut butter (crunchy or smooth), 2 tablespoons natural

Meal Building Block Swaps

Swap any of the same category foods in each row for one another. I've listed only the foods that show up in your 28-day plan, but you can feel free to incorporate foods you don't see in your meal plan, such as sweet potatoes, eggplant, kiwifruit, celery, etc. The list goes on and on! Again, consult the Eat These Foods Regularly and Eat These Foods Sparingly lists at the back of the book for serving sizes and calorie counts to make swapping easy.

BUILDING BLOCK	FOODS
Lean Protein	Canned wild salmon Cannellini beans Chunk light water-pack tuna Egg whites (or egg substitutes) Frozen meatless chicken-style nuggets Hummus Kidney beans Organic deli chicken breast* Organic deli roast beef* Organic deli turkey breast* Veggie burgers
Dairy	Fat-free cottage cheese Fat-free milk Fat-free ricotta cheese Fat-free yogurt** Light or low-fat string cheese*** Reduced-fat Cheddar cheese Reduced-fat Monterey Jack cheese Reduced-fat shredded mozzarella cheese
Fruits	Apples Bananas Blueberries, fresh or frozen unsweetened Dried cranberries, unsweetened Grapefruit Mangoes, fresh or frozen unsweetened Oranges Peaches, fresh or frozen unsweetened Pears Pineapple tidbits, canned in 100% pineapple juice Red or green grapes Strawberries, fresh or frozen unsweetened

BUILDING BLOCK	FOODS
Vegetables	Baby carrots Baby spinach leaves Bell peppers Frozen Chinese-style vegetables (includes any combination of bamboo shoots, broccoli, carrots, cauliflower, mushrooms, onions, water chestnuts) Mixed baby greens Onions Romaine lettuce Tomatoes
Breads, Cereals, and Grains	Brown rice Rolled oats (oatmeal) Whole grain cereal Whole wheat bread Whole wheat crackers Whole wheat English muffins Whole wheat pasta Whole wheat pita Whole wheat wraps
Spices, Seasonings, and Condiments	Balsamic vinegar Canola oil mayonnaise Dijon mustard Dried herbs and spices Fresh herbs Lemon juice Lime juice

*We call for organic deli meat because it is generally lower in sodium and fat. If you choose to purchase nonorganic meat, please look for low-sodium choices.

**Because many fat-free yogurts contain artificial flavorings and sweeteners, please be careful about the brands you choose and read the label carefully!

***We call for light or low-fat string cheese rather than part-skim because it is lower in saturated fat and calories. If you have trouble finding light or low-fat string cheese, though, feel free to substitute with part-skim string cheese.

SHOPPING MADE EASY

Your Ultimate 28-Day Eating Plan is designed to save you time and money. We've carefully planned the meals so that you will be able to use all of the perishable foods you buy each week (that means no waste), plus we'll help you reuse dry goods and frozen foods throughout the entire plan.

Bear in mind that this means your shopping list in Week 1 is a little longer than it is for the rest of the plan. That's because all of the pantry items—condiments, canned foods, oils, bread products, bars, frozen foods, and nuts—that you'll need for all 28 days are included. You may already have a lot of these items on hand, but just in case you don't, you should make a big stock-up trip to a discount grocery store. Having these essentials handy will make it easier to stay on the *Flat Belly Diet* for the full 28 days.

Keep perishable bread products in the freezer—they'll keep for at least 3 months. Let them defrost on the counter before using them, or if you're in a hurry, place in the microwave on the defrost setting for about a minute. Store nuts in the freezer or refrigerator (see page 27). When using nuts or seeds in meals, measure them whole, then chop them up for meals.

One final note: Your Ultimate 28-Day Eating Plan was designed for one person, so all of the recipes and shopping lists include just enough food for one. If you're following this plan with your spouse or a roommate, double the amounts. We always tell you how much of each ingredient you'll be using in each week and, in weeks 2, 3, and 4, which ingredients should be left over from the previous week(s) if you were following the plan exactly. (You'll see some frozen and dry goods in Week 1 without an indication of how much you'll be using; those are foods you won't need until later in the plan.)

Note: For dairy or other fresh items that you purchase from week to week, please check the use-by date to be sure they will take you through the whole week.

Note: Fresh herbs are included in some of these recipes. If you need to substitute dried herbs, use one-third of the suggested amount.

Note: Purchasing small amounts of vegetables from the grocery salad bar may save you time and money.

DAY	MEAL	RECIPE	MUFA
1	Breakfast	Pumpkin Crunch Cereal	Pumpkin seeds
1	Lunch	Chicken and Apple Salad	Olive oil
1	Snack Pack	Strawberry Chocolate Waffle	Dark chocolate
1	Dinner	Guacamole Dip	Hass avocado
2	Breakfast	Walnut Apple Waffle	Walnuts
2	Lunch	Chicken Sandwich	Hass avocado
2	Snack Pack	Apples and Crackers	Almond butter
2	Dinner	Scrambled Egg with Toast	Hass avocado
3	Breakfast	Mango Strawberry Smoothie	Almond butter
3	Lunch	California Burger	Hass avocado
3	Snack Pack	Fruit and Nuts	Walnuts
3	Dinner	Dijon Salmon Pita	Pumpkin seeds
4	Breakfast	**Walnut Apple Waffle**	Walnuts
4	Lunch	Avocado and Salmon Salad	Hass avocado
4	Snack Pack	**Strawberry Chocolate Waffle**	Dark chocolate
4	Dinner	Waldorf Pita	Walnuts
5	Breakfast	**Mango Strawberry Smoothie**	Almond butter
5	Lunch	**Chicken and Apple Salad**	Olive oil
5	Snack Pack	**Fruit and Nuts**	Walnuts
5	Dinner	**Guacamole Dip**	Hass avocado
6	Breakfast	**Pumpkin Crunch Cereal**	Pumpkin seeds
6	Lunch	**California Burger**	Hass avocado
6	Snack Pack	**Apples and Crackers**	Almond butter
6	Dinner	Chicken Herb Crackers	Walnuts
7	Breakfast	**Mango Strawberry Smoothie**	Almond butter
7	Lunch	**Avocado and Salmon Salad**	Hass avocado
7	Snack Pack	String Cheese and Fruit Cup	Peanuts
7	Dinner	**Waldorf Pita**	Walnuts

Bold = Repeated Recipe

SHOPPING LIST

PRODUCE

- Apples, any type, 8 medium (using 8)
- Granny Smith apples, 2 medium (using 2)
- Bananas, 5 small (using 5)
- Grapefruit, 3 (using 3)
- Mangoes, 2 fresh or frozen unsweetened chunks, 10-ounce bag (using 10 ounces)
- Strawberries, 18 ounces fresh or frozen unsweetened, 2 (10-ounce) packages (using $3\frac{1}{2}$ cups or 18 ounces)
- Hass avocados, 4 small (using 4)
- Baby carrots, 4-ounce package (1 cup) (using 1 cup)
- Cucumber, 1 small (using 1)
- Romaine lettuce, 3 (10-ounce) packages (using 3 packages)
- Red bell peppers, 3 medium (using 3)
- Tomatoes, 7 small (using 7)
- Orange juice, 100% pure, 1 quart
- Cilantro, 1 small bunch fresh (optional) (using 1)
- Parsley, 1 small bunch fresh (optional) (using 1)
- Tarragon, 1 small bunch fresh (optional) (using 1)

DAIRY

- Fat-free milk, $\frac{1}{2}$ gallon (using 5 cups)
- Laughing Cow Light Garlic & Herb Wedges, 6-ounce package (using 5 wedges)
- String cheese, 6-ounce package light or low-fat (using 3 pieces)* (If you are starting this plan immediately after doing the 4-day jumpstart, you should have 2 pieces string cheese left over to use this week.)

EGGS

- Liquid egg whites, 8-ounce container (using $\frac{1}{2}$ cup)

FROZEN FOODS

- Whole grain frozen waffles, 1 package (using 6)
- Whole cut corn, no salt added, 10-ounce package frozen
- Edamame (soybeans), 2 (10-ounce) packages frozen shelled
- Stir-fry or Chinese-style frozen vegetables (may include broccoli, carrots, cauliflower, mushrooms, water chestnuts; but if this mixture is not available, select a similar mixture), 2 (10-ounce) packages
- Meatless chicken-style nuggets, 2 (12-ounce) boxes
- Veggie burgers, 2 (4-count) packages, (using 2)

BREAD/CEREAL

- Whole wheat bread, 1-pound loaf, 16 slices (using 4 slices)
- Whole wheat pita pockets, about 6" diameter, 1 (8-count) package (using 7)
- Whole wheat wraps, 8" diameter, 1 (6-count) package

Whole wheat crackers, about 1½″ square, 12-ounce box (using 42)

Rolled oats, 18-ounce canister

Kashi 7 Whole Grain Puffs, 12-ounce box (using 2 cups)

DRY GOODS

Canola oil, 8-ounce bottle

Flaxseed oil, 8-ounce bottle cold-pressed (If you are starting this plan immediately after doing the 4-day jump-start, you should have enough flaxseed oil to take you through the 28-day plan and don't need to buy any more.)

Extra virgin olive oil, 8-ounce bottle (using 3 tablespoons plus 1 teaspoon) (If you are starting this plan immediately after doing the 4-day jumpstart, you should have enough olive oil to take you through the 28-day plan and don't need to buy more.)

High-oleic safflower oil, 8-ounce bottle

Sesame oil, 6-ounce bottle

Sunflower oil, 8-ounce bottle

Almond butter, 8-ounce jar (using 10 tablespoons)

Almonds, 8-ounce package roasted or raw unsalted

Brazil nuts, 6-ounce package roasted or raw unsalted

Hazelnuts, ¼ cup bulk (or 2-ounce package) raw or roasted unsalted

Macadamia nuts, ¼ cup bulk (or 2-ounce package) raw unsalted

Pecans, 1 cup bulk (or 8-ounce package) roasted or raw unsalted

Pine nuts, 6-ounce package roasted or raw unsalted

Pistachios, ½ cup bulk (or 4-ounce package) raw unsalted

Walnut halves, 6-ounce package raw unsalted (using 14 tablespoons)

Peanut butter, natural, 12-ounce jar

Peanuts, ⅛ cup bulk (or 2-ounce package), roasted or raw unsalted (using 2 tablespoons)

Pumpkin seeds, ½ cup bulk (or 8-ounce package), roasted or raw unsalted (using 6 tablespoons)

Sesame seeds, 2 tablespoons or ¾ ounce

Sunflower seeds, ½ cup bulk (or 3-ounce package) raw unsalted

Cannellini beans, no salt added, 15-ounce can

Kidney beans, no salt added, 15-ounce can

Green olives, 15-ounce jar large

Black olives, 15-ounce can plus 7-ounce can large

Semisweet or dark chocolate chips, 12-ounce package (using ½ cup)

Cranberries, dried, unsweetened, 8-ounce package

SHOPPING LIST—CONT.

DRY GOODS (CONT.)

Raisins, seedless, 15-ounce container (If you are starting this plan immediately after doing the 4-day jumpstart, you should have enough raisins to take you through the 28-day plan and don't need to buy any more.)

Pineapple tidbits, packed in juice, 20-ounce can plus 8-ounce can (or eight 4-ounce cups) (using 4 ounces)

Roasted red peppers, 12-ounce jar

Dijon mustard, 8-ounce or smaller jar (using 4 teaspoons)

Canola oil mayonnaise, 8-ounce jar

Agave nectar, 1 small bottle (using 4 teaspoons)

Chicken broth, reduced-sodium, 2 (16-ounce) cans

Marinara sauce with less than 400 milligrams of sodium per $\frac{1}{2}$-cup serving, 8-ounce jar

MEAL REPLACEMENT BARS

Choose 7 of any of the following meal replacement bars. These bars are interchangeable on the plan wherever you see a bar listed with a meal or snack.

Luna: Chai Tea, Chocolate Pecan Pie, or Lemon Zest Bar

Nature's Path: Optimum Energy Bar Blueberry Flax & Soy or Pomegran Cherry

MEAT/SEAFOOD

Wild salmon, 6-ounce can, or 8 ounces fresh salmon (using 6 ounces) (If you prefer to bake or broil your own salmon for these meals, purchase 3 ounces raw salmon for each 2 ounces cooked salmon in your meals. The raw weight for fish and meat is a little more than the cooked weight.)

Chunk light water-pack tuna, 4 (3-ounce) cans (or two 6-ounce cans) or fresh or frozen tuna steak, 14 ounces (divide into $3\frac{1}{2}$-ounce portions, store in freezer, defrost, and cook as needed)

Organic deli chicken breast, 12-ounce package (using 12 ounces)**

SPICES AND SEASONINGS

Ginger, ground, 1-ounce container

Basil, dried, 1-ounce container

Balsamic vinegar, aged, 8-ounce bottle (using 4 tablespoons)

Rice vinegar, 6-ounce bottle (using 2 tablespoons)

Sherry vinegar, 6-ounce bottle

*We call for light or low-fat string cheese rather than part-skim because it is lower in saturated fat and calories. If you have trouble finding light or low-fat string cheese, though, feel free to substitute with part-skim string cheese.

**We call for organic deli meat because it is generally lower in sodium and fat. If you choose to purchase nonorganic meat, please look for low-sodium choices.

DAY 1

Pumpkin Crunch Cereal: Mix 1 cup Kashi 7 Whole Grain Puffs (75) with 1 cup fat-free milk (80) and 1 small banana, sliced (90); top with 2 tablespoons **pumpkin seeds** (148).

Total calories: 393

Chicken and Apple Salad: Mix 3 cups shredded romaine lettuce (24), 1 small tomato, sliced (12), 1 medium tart apple (such as Granny Smith), diced (95), and 3 ounces organic deli chicken breast, sliced into small pieces (75). Toss with 1 tablespoon **olive oil** (119) and 2 tablespoons balsamic vinegar (10). Crumble 2 small whole wheat crackers over top (36).

Total calories: 371

Strawberry Chocolate Waffle: Top 1 frozen whole grain waffle (100) with $\frac{1}{4}$ cup **semisweet or dark chocolate chips** (207) and place in a toaster oven or oven set to 350°F for 2 minutes to toast the waffle and slightly melt the chocolate chips. Top with 1 cup fresh or thawed frozen unsweetened strawberries (52).

Total calories: 359

Guacamole Dip: Toast 1 whole wheat pita (140) and cut or break into triangles; dip into a mixture of $\frac{1}{4}$ cup chopped **Hass avocado** (96), 1 teaspoon agave nectar (20), 1 teaspoon chopped cilantro leaves (0), 2 small tomatoes, chopped (24), and $\frac{1}{2}$ cup finely chopped red bell pepper (23). Have 1 light or low-fat string cheese (80).

Total calories: 383

DAY 2

Walnut Apple Waffle: Toast 2 frozen whole grain waffles (200) and top with a mixture of 1 medium apple, chopped (95), 1 teaspoon agave nectar (20), and 2 tablespoons **walnuts** (82).

Total calories: 397

LUNCH

Chicken Sandwich: Spread 2 slices whole wheat bread (160) with ¼ cup sliced ripe **Hass avocado,** mashed (96); fill with 3 ounces organic deli chicken breast (75), ½ cup shredded romaine lettuce (4), and 1 teaspoon chopped fresh tarragon (0). Have 1 small banana (90).

Total calories: 425

SNACK PACK

Apples and Crackers: Spread 6 small whole wheat crackers (108) with 2 tablespoons **almond butter** (200) and serve with 1 medium apple (95).

Total calories: 403

DINNER

Scrambled Egg with Toast: Toast 2 slices whole wheat bread (160) and top with ¼ cup sliced **Hass avocado** (96) and 1 small tomato, sliced (12). Scramble ½ cup egg whites (50) with cooking spray, with salt and pepper to taste. Have ½ grapefruit (60).

Total calories: 378

DAY 3

Mango Strawberry Smoothie: In a blender, combine 1 cup fat-free milk (80), 2 tablespoons **almond butter** (200), 1/2 cup fresh or frozen unsweetened strawberries (26), and 1/2 cup fresh or frozen unsweetened mango chunks (60).

Total calories: 366

California Burger: Fill 1 whole wheat pita (140) with 1 cooked veggie burger (100) dressed with 1 teaspoon Dijon mustard (5); add 1/2 cup shredded romaine lettuce (4), 1/2 cup sliced red bell pepper (23), and 1/4 cup sliced **Hass avocado** (96).

Total calories: 368

Fruit and Nuts: Mix 1 medium apple, diced (95), 1 small banana, sliced (90), and 2 tablespoons orange juice (14). Top with 2 tablespoons **walnuts** (82). Have 6 small whole wheat crackers (108).

Total calories: 389

Dijon Salmon Pita: Spread 1 whole wheat pita (140) with 2 teaspoons Dijon mustard (10) and sprinkle with 2 tablespoons **pumpkin seeds** (148), 1 teaspoon chopped fresh parsley (0), and 1/4 cucumber, thinly sliced (9). Fill with 2 ounces canned wild salmon (90).

Total calories: 397

DAY 4

BREAKFAST

Walnut Apple Waffle: Toast 2 frozen whole grain waffles (200) and top with a mixture of 1 medium apple, chopped (95), 1 teaspoon agave nectar (20), and 2 tablespoons **walnuts** (82).

Total calories: 397

LUNCH

Avocado and Salmon Salad: Mix 3 cups shredded romaine lettuce (24), 2 ounces canned wild salmon (90), 1 grapefruit, sectioned and sliced (120), $\frac{1}{4}$ cup chopped **Hass avocado** (96), 1 tablespoon rice vinegar (0), and 2 teaspoons olive oil (79).

Total calories: 409

SNACK PACK

Strawberry Chocolate Waffle: Top 1 frozen whole grain waffle (100) with $\frac{1}{4}$ cup **semisweet or dark chocolate chips** (207) and place in a toaster oven or oven set to 350°F for 2 minutes to toast the waffle and slightly melt the chocolate chips. Top with 1 cup fresh or thawed frozen unsweetened strawberries (52).

Total calories: 359

DINNER

Waldorf Pita: Split 1 whole wheat pita (140), spread with 2 Laughing Cow Light Garlic & Herb Wedges (70), and fill with 1 medium apple, chopped (95), 2 tablespoons **walnuts** (82), and 1 cup shredded romaine lettuce (8).

Total calories: 395

DAY 5

BREAKFAST

Mango Strawberry Smoothie: In a blender, combine 1 cup fat-free milk (80), 2 tablespoons **almond butter** (200), $\frac{1}{2}$ cup fresh or frozen unsweetened strawberries (26), and $\frac{1}{2}$ cup fresh or frozen unsweetened mango chunks (60).

Total calories: 366

LUNCH

Chicken and Apple Salad: Mix 3 cups shredded romaine lettuce (24), 1 small tomato, sliced (12), 1 medium tart apple (such as Granny Smith), diced (95), and 3 ounces organic deli chicken breast, sliced into small pieces (75). Toss with 1 tablespoon **olive oil** (119) and 2 tablespoons balsamic vinegar (10). Crumble 2 small whole wheat crackers over top (36).

Total calories: 371

SNACK PACK

Fruit and Nuts: Mix 1 medium apple, diced (95), 1 small banana, sliced (90), and 2 tablespoons orange juice (14). Top with 2 tablespoons **walnuts** (82). Have 6 small whole wheat crackers (108).

Total calories: 389

DINNER

Guacamole Dip: Toast 1 whole wheat pita (140) and cut into triangles; dip into a mixture of $\frac{1}{4}$ cup chopped **Hass avocado** (96), 1 teaspoon agave nectar (20), 1 teaspoon chopped cilantro leaves (0), 2 small tomatoes, chopped (24), and $\frac{1}{2}$ cup finely chopped red bell pepper (23). Have 1 light or low-fat string cheese (80).

Total calories: 383

DAY 6

BREAKFAST

Pumpkin Crunch Cereal: Mix 1 cup Kashi 7 Whole Grain Puffs (75) with 1 cup fat-free milk (80) and 1 small banana, sliced (90); top with 2 tablespoons **pumpkin seeds** (148).

Total calories: 393

LUNCH

California Burger: Fill 1 whole wheat pita (140) with 1 cooked veggie burger (100) dressed with 1 teaspoon Dijon mustard (5); add $\frac{1}{2}$ cup shredded romaine lettuce (4), $\frac{1}{2}$ cup sliced red bell pepper (23), and $\frac{1}{4}$ cup chopped **Hass avocado** (96).

Total calories: 368

SNACK PACK

Apples and Crackers: Spread 6 small whole wheat crackers (108) with 2 tablespoons **almond butter** (200). Have 1 medium apple (95).

Total calories: 403

DINNER

Chicken Herb Crackers: Spread 8 small whole wheat crackers (144) with 1 Laughing Cow Light Garlic & Herb Wedge (35) and top with 3 ounces organic deli chicken breast, cubed (75). Have $\frac{1}{2}$ cup sliced mango (60) topped with 2 tablespoons **walnuts** (82).

Total calories: 396

DAY 7

BREAKFAST

Mango Strawberry Smoothie: In a blender, combine 1 cup fat-free milk (80), 2 tablespoons **almond butter** (200), $\frac{1}{2}$ cup fresh or frozen unsweetened strawberries (26), and $\frac{1}{2}$ cup fresh or frozen unsweetened mango chunks (60).

Total calories: 366

LUNCH

Avocado and Salmon Salad: Mix 3 cups shredded romaine lettuce (24), 2 ounces canned wild salmon (90), 1 grapefruit, sectioned and sliced (120), $\frac{1}{4}$ cup chopped **Hass avocado** (96), 1 tablespoon rice vinegar (0), and 2 teaspoons olive oil (79).

Total calories: 409

SNACK PACK

String Cheese and Fruit Cup: Have 1 light or low-fat string cheese (60), 4 ounces pineapple tidbits canned in juice (60), 1 cup baby carrots (50), 6 small whole wheat crackers (108), and 2 tablespoons **peanuts** (110).

Total calories: 388

DINNER

Waldorf Pita: Split 1 whole wheat pita (140), spread with 2 Laughing Cow Light Garlic & Herb Wedges (70), and fill with 1 medium apple, chopped (95), 2 tablespoons **walnuts** (82), and 1 cup shredded romaine lettuce (8).

Total calories: 395

DAY	MEAL	RECIPE	MUFA
8	Breakfast	Vanilla Pecan Parfait	Pecans
8	Lunch	Sesame Chicken Stir-Fry	Sesame oil
8	Snack Pack	Bar and Sunflower Seeds	Sunflower seeds
8	Dinner	Mediterranean Sandwich	Pine nuts
9	Breakfast	Sweet and Savory Cottage Cheese	Pine nuts
9	Lunch	Edamame Potato Salad	Edamame
9	Snack Pack	Yogurt and Pecans	Pecans
9	Dinner	Tapenade Pasta	Black olive tapenade
10	Breakfast	Cranberry Hazelnut Cereal	Hazelnuts
10	Lunch	Red Pepper Tapenade Wrap	Black olive tapenade
10	Snack Pack	Hummus Dip	Pine nuts
10	Dinner	Baby Green Pocket	Pecans
11	Breakfast	**Vanilla Pecan Parfait**	Pecans
11	Lunch	Chinese Chicken	Sesame oil
11	Snack Pack	Cheese and Crackers	Sunflower seeds
11	Dinner	Tuna Salad	Pine nuts
12	Breakfast	**Sweet and Savory Cottage Cheese**	Pine nuts
12	Lunch	**Red Pepper Tapenade Wrap**	Black olive tapenade
12	Snack Pack	**Bar and Sunflower Seeds**	Sunflower seeds
12	Dinner	Edamame Stir-Fry	Edamame
13	Breakfast	**Cranberry Hazelnut Cereal**	Hazelnuts
13	Lunch	**Sesame Chicken Stir-Fry**	Sesame oil
13	Snack Pack	**Hummus Dip**	Pine nuts
13	Dinner	**Tapenade Pasta**	Black olive tapenade
14	Breakfast	**Sweet and Savory Cottage Cheese**	Pine nuts
14	Lunch	**Edamame Potato Salad**	Edamame
14	Snack Pack	**Cheese and Crackers**	Sunflower seeds
14	Dinner	**Baby Green Pocket**	Pecans

Bold = Repeated Recipe

SHOPPING LIST

Note: Beginning this week, you'll notice some items listed in *italics.* If you've been following this plan exactly, you purchased these items in week 1 and should have enough of this food to fulfill what you need this week for the meal plan. We've added this information here just in case you're short on any ingredients for any reason.

PRODUCE

Navel oranges, 8 medium (using 8)

Red or green grapes, 2½ pounds (using 2½ pounds)

Raspberries, 10 ounces fresh or 10-ounce package frozen unsweetened (using 10 ounces)

Baby greens, 10-ounce package mixed (using 1 package)

Baby spinach leaves, 2 (10-ounce) packages (using 2 packages)

Red bell peppers, 2 medium (using 2)

Red potatoes, 2 (3½-ounce) (using 2)

Scallions, 1 small bunch (if possible, from the salad bar) (using 5)

Lemon, 1 (using 1)

Parsley, fresh, 1 bunch (optional) (using 1)

DAIRY

Fat-free milk, 1 quart (using 4 cups)

Fat-free vanilla yogurt, 3 (6-ounce) containers

Fat-free cottage cheese, 2 (16-ounce) containers (using 3 cups)

Mozzarella cheese, 8-ounce package shredded reduced-fat (using 6 tablespoons)

String cheese, 6-ounce package light or low-fat (using 2 pieces)*

FROZEN FOODS

Frozen whole cut corn, no salt added (using 1 cup)

Frozen shelled edamame (soybeans) (using 3 cups)

Stir-fry or Chinese-style frozen vegetables (may include broccoli, carrots, cauliflower, mushrooms, water chestnuts; if this mixture is not available, select a similar mixture) (using 3 cups)

Meatless chicken-style nuggets (using 9)

Veggie burgers (using 2)

SHOPPING LIST—CONT.

BREAD/CEREAL

Whole wheat bread
(using 2 slices)

Whole wheat wraps
(using 2)

Whole wheat pita pockets,
about 6" diameter, 1 (8-count)
package (using 2)

Whole wheat crackers,
about 1½" square (using 24)

Kashi 7 Whole Grain Puffs
(using 5 cups)

Whole wheat pasta,
any shape (using 1½ cups
cooked)

Brown rice (If you are
starting the plan immediately
after doing the 4-day
jumpstart, you should
have enough.) (using ½ cup
cooked)

DRY GOODS

Olive oil (using 1 tablespoon
plus 1 teaspoon)

Hazelnuts, raw or roasted
unsalted (using ¼ cup)

Sesame oil (using
3 tablespoons)

Pecans, roasted or
raw unsalted (using
10 tablespoons)

Pine nuts, roasted or
raw unsalted (using
14 tablespoons)

Sunflower seeds, raw
unsalted (using
8 tablespoons)

Sesame seeds (using
2 tablespoons)

Cranberries, dried
unsweetened (using
4 tablespoons)

Roasted red peppers, jarred
(using 1 cup)

Canola oil mayonnaise
(using 3 teaspoons)

MEAL REPLACEMENT BARS

Luna: Chai Tea, Chocolate
Pecan Pie, or Lemon Zest Bar
or Nature's Path: Optimum
Energy Bar Blueberry Flax
& Soy or Pomegran Cherry
(using 2)

MEAT/SEAFOOD

Chunk light water-pack
tuna or 12 ounces fresh
or frozen tuna steak (using
6 ounces)

SPICES AND SEASONINGS

☐ *Balsamic vinegar (using 1 tablespoon)*

☐ *Rice vinegar (using 5 tablespoons plus 2 teaspoons)*

☐ Hummus, 8-ounce container (using 1 cup)

☐ Olive tapenade, 4.6-ounce container (You should be able to find this in the refrigerated section near the hummus or deli-style olives, or ask your store manager.) (using 8 tablespoons)

*We call for light or low-fat string cheese rather than part-skim because it is lower in saturated fat and calories. If you have trouble finding light or low-fat string cheese, though, feel free to substitute with part-skim string cheese.

DAY 8

BREAKFAST

Vanilla Pecan Parfait: Layer half of these ingredients in this order in a parfait glass; repeat layers, ending with pecans: 1 cup Kashi 7 Whole Grain Puffs (70), 1 cup fresh or thawed frozen unsweetened raspberries (70), 6 ounces fat-free vanilla yogurt (155), and 2 tablespoons **pecans** (90).

Total calories: 385

LUNCH

Sesame Chicken Stir-Fry: Stir-fry 3 cups baby spinach leaves (24) in 1 tablespoon toasted **sesame oil** (120), 2 tablespoons rice vinegar (0), and 1 tablespoon sesame seeds (51) for 2 to 3 minutes. Cook 3 meatless chicken-style nuggets (129) in the microwave according to package directions and add to the mixture; toss to combine and heat for 1 minute. Serve with 1 medium orange (62).

Total calories: 386

SNACK PACK

Bar and Sunflower Seeds: Have 1 Nature's Path Optimum Blueberry Flax & Soy or Pomegran Cherry bar (200), 2 tablespoons **sunflower seeds** (90), and 1 medium orange, sliced (62).

Total calories: 352

DINNER

Mediterranean Sandwich: Mix 3 ounces canned chunk light water-pack tuna, drained (105), with 1 teaspoon canola oil mayonnaise (33), 1 tablespoon rice vinegar (0), 1 teaspoon chopped fresh parsley (0), 1 teaspoon lemon juice (1), and 2 tablespoons **pine nuts** (113). Fill 2 slices whole wheat bread (160) with the tuna mixture.

Total calories: 412

DAY 9

Sweet and Savory Cottage Cheese: Mix 1 cup fat-free cottage cheese (180), 2 tablespoons toasted **pine nuts** (113), and 1 cup red or green grapes, sliced (104).

Total calories: 397

Edamame Potato Salad: Combine 1 cup shelled and boiled **edamame** (298) with a boiled, then chopped 3-ounce red potato (skin on) (74), 1 teaspoon rice vinegar (0), 1 teaspoon canola oil mayonnaise (33), and 2 scallions, thinly sliced (10). Season with black pepper.

Total calories: 415

Yogurt and Pecans: Have 6 ounces fat-free vanilla yogurt (155) topped with 2 tablespoons **pecans** (90). Have 1 cup red or green grapes (104).

Total calories: 349

Tapenade Pasta: Mix ³/₄ cup cooked whole wheat pasta, any shape (131), 2 tablespoons **black olive tapenade** (88), 2 teaspoons olive oil (79), 3 tablespoons shredded reduced-fat mozzarella cheese (52), and ¹/₄ cup roasted red peppers (12). Microwave to warm through and melt the cheese.

Total calories: 362

DAY 10

Cranberry Hazelnut Cereal: Mix 1½ cups Kashi 7 Whole Grain Puffs (105), 1 cup fat-free milk (80), 2 tablespoons **hazelnuts** (110), and 2 tablespoons dried cranberries (45). Have 1 medium orange (62).

Total calories: 402

LUNCH

Red Pepper Tapenade Wrap: Spread 1 whole wheat wrap (140) with 2 tablespoons **black olive tapenade** (88) and fill with ¼ cup roasted red peppers (12). Have 1 cup fat-free milk (80) and 1 medium orange (62).

Total calories: 382

SNACK PACK

Hummus Dip: Dip 1 cup sliced red bell peppers (46) into ½ cup hummus (200) sprinkled with 2 tablespoons **pine nuts** (113).

Total calories: 359

DINNER

Baby Green Pocket: Fill 1 whole wheat pita (140) with a mixture of 1 cooked and crumbled veggie burger (100), 1 cup mixed baby greens (9), ½ cup cooked corn (66), and 2 tablespoons **pecans** (90).

Total calories: 405

DAY 11

BREAKFAST

Vanilla Pecan Parfait: Layer half of these ingredients in this order in a parfait glass; repeat layers, ending with pecans: 1 cup Kashi 7 Whole Grain Puffs (70), 1 cup fresh or thawed frozen unsweetened raspberries (70), 6 ounces fat-free vanilla yogurt (155), and 2 tablespoons **pecans** (90).

Total calories: 385

LUNCH

Chinese Chicken: Heat 2 cups frozen Chinese-style vegetables (52) with 1 tablespoon **sesame oil** (120); serve with 3 cooked meatless chicken-style nuggets (129) and $\frac{1}{2}$ cup cooked brown rice (109).

Total calories: 410

SNACK PACK

Cheese and Crackers: Have 1 light or low-fat string cheese (60), 8 small whole wheat crackers (144), and 2 tablespoons **sunflower seeds** (90). Have 1 cup red or green grapes (104).

Total calories: 398

DINNER

Tuna Salad: Mix 2 cups baby spinach leaves (16), 1 tablespoon lemon juice (3), 1 teaspoon chopped fresh parsley (0), and 1 tablespoon balsamic vinegar (10); top with 3 ounces canned chunk light water-pack tuna (105) and 2 tablespoons **pine nuts** (113). Have 8 small whole wheat crackers (144).

Total calories: 391

DAY 12

BREAKFAST

Sweet and Savory Cottage Cheese: Mix 1 cup fat-free cottage cheese (180), 2 tablespoons toasted **pine nuts** (113), and 1 cup red or green grapes, sliced (104).

Total calories: 397

LUNCH

Red Pepper Tapenade Wrap: Spread 1 whole wheat wrap (140) with 2 tablespoons **black olive tapenade** (88) and fill with ¼ cup roasted red peppers (12). Have 1 cup fat-free milk (80) and 1 medium orange (62).

Total calories: 382

SNACK PACK

Bar and Sunflower Seeds: Have 1 Nature's Path Optimum Blueberry Flax & Soy or Pomegran Cherry bar (200), 2 tablespoons **sunflower seeds** (90), and 1 medium orange, sliced (62).

Total calories: 352

DINNER

Edamame Stir-Fry: In a medium skillet, heat 1 teaspoon sesame oil (40), 1 scallion, sliced (5), 1 cup shelled and boiled **edamame** (298), and 1 cup frozen Chinese-style vegetables (26).

Total calories: 369

DAY 13

BREAKFAST

Cranberry Hazelnut Cereal: Mix 1½ cups Kashi 7 Whole Grain Puffs (105), 1 cup fat-free milk (80), 2 tablespoons **hazelnuts** (110), and 2 tablespoons dried cranberries (45). Have 1 medium orange (62).

Total calories: 402

LUNCH

Sesame Chicken Stir-Fry: Stir-fry 3 cups baby spinach leaves (24) in 1 tablespoon toasted **sesame oil** (120), 2 tablespoons rice vinegar (0), and 1 tablespoon sesame seeds (51) for 2 to 3 minutes. Cook 3 meatless chicken-style nuggets (129) in the microwave according to package directions and add to the mixture; toss to combine and heat for 1 minute. Serve with 1 medium orange (62).

Total calories: 386

SNACK PACK

Hummus Dip: Dip 1 cup sliced red bell peppers (46) into ½ cup hummus (200) sprinkled with 2 tablespoons **pine nuts** (113).

Total calories: 359

DINNER

Tapenade Pasta: Mix ¾ cup cooked whole wheat pasta, any shape (131), 2 tablespoons **black olive tapenade** (88), 2 teaspoons olive oil (79), 3 tablespoons shredded reduced-fat mozzarella cheese (52), and ¼ cup roasted red peppers (12). Microwave to warm through and melt the cheese.

Total calories: 362

DAY 14

BREAKFAST

Sweet and Savory Cottage Cheese: Mix 1 cup fat-free cottage cheese (180), 2 tablespoons toasted **pine nuts** (113), and 1 cup red or green grapes, sliced (104).

Total calories: 397

LUNCH

Edamame Potato Salad: Combine 1 cup shelled and boiled **edamame** (298) with a boiled, then chopped 3-ounce red potato (skin on) (74), 1 teaspoon rice vinegar (0), 1 teaspoon canola oil mayonnaise (33), and 2 scallions, thinly sliced (10). Season with black pepper.

Total calories: 415

SNACK PACK

Cheese and Crackers: Have 1 light or low-fat string cheese (60), 8 small whole wheat crackers (144), and 2 tablespoons **sunflower seeds** (90). Have 1 cup red or green grapes (104).

Total calories: 398

DINNER

Baby Green Pocket: Fill 1 whole wheat pita (140) with a mixture of 1 cooked and crumbled veggie burger (100), 1 cup mixed baby greens (9), ½ cup cooked corn (66), and 2 tablespoons **pecans** (90).

Total calories: 405

DAY	MEAL	RECIPE	MUFA
15	Breakfast	Bar and Chocolate Chips	Dark chocolate
15	Lunch	Picnic Lunch	Green olives
15	Snack Pack	Crackers and Peanut Butter	Peanut butter
15	Dinner	White Bean Pasta	Pesto
16	Breakfast	Raisin and Nut Cereal	Almonds
16	Lunch	Peanutty Cranberry Wrap	Peanut butter
16	Snack Pack	Deli Snack	Black olive tapenade
16	Dinner	Basil Bean Salad	Olive oil
17	Breakfast	Peach Almond Oatmeal	Almonds
17	Lunch	Creamy Peanut Soup	Peanut butter
17	Snack Pack	Olive and Provolone Sandwich	Green olives
17	Dinner	Veggie Pita	Sunflower oil
18	Breakfast	**Bar and Chocolate Chips**	Dark chocolate
18	Lunch	**Picnic Lunch**	Green olives
18	Snack Pack	Yogurt and Brazil Nuts	Brazil nuts
18	Dinner	Spinach Sunflower Stir-Fry	Sunflower oil
19	Breakfast	**Raisin and Nut Cereal**	Almonds
19	Lunch	**Cranberry Nut Ricotta Dip**	Brazil nuts
19	Snack Pack	**Olive and Provolone Sandwich**	Green olives
19	Dinner	**White Bean Pasta**	Pesto
20	Breakfast	**Peach Almond Oatmeal**	Almonds
20	Lunch	**Peanutty Cranberry Wrap**	Peanut butter
20	Snack Pack	**Yogurt and Brazil Nuts**	Brazil nuts
20	Dinner	Cheesy Pasta with Spinach	Canola oil
21	Breakfast	**Bar and Chocolate Chips**	Dark chocolate
21	Lunch	**Creamy Peanut Soup**	Peanut butter
21	Snack Pack	**Deli Snack**	Black olive tapenade
21	Dinner	**Veggie Pita**	Sunflower oil

Bold = Repeated Recipe

SHOPPING LIST

Note: You'll notice some items listed in *italics*. If you've been following this plan exactly, you purchased these items in week 1 and should have enough of this food to fulfill what you need this week for the meal plan. We've added this information here just in case you're short on any ingredients for any reason.

PRODUCE

Oranges, 5 (using 5)

Peaches, 10 ounces fresh sliced (about 2 medium peaches) or 10-ounce package frozen unsweetened sliced (using 10 ounces)

Baby carrots, 24-ounce package (using 1 package)

Celery, ½ cup diced (if possible, from the salad bar) or 1 small bunch celery (using ½ cup)

Baby greens, 10-ounce package mixed (using 1 package)

Baby spinach leaves, 10-ounce package (using 1 package)

Lemon, 1 (using 1)

Garlic, 1 small head (using 1)

White or yellow onion, 1 small (using 1)

Parsley, 1 small bunch (optional) (using 1)

Tomato, 1 small (using 1)

DAIRY

Fat-free milk, ½ gallon (using 4 cups)

Fat-free vanilla yogurt, 2 (6-ounce) containers

Laughing Cow Light Garlic & Herb Wedges, 1 package (using 4 wedges)

Mozzarella cheese, shredded reduced-fat (using 3 tablespoons)

Provolone cheese, 2 ounces sliced reduced-fat

Ricotta cheese, 15-ounce container fat-free (using 1 cup)

String cheese, 6-ounce package light or low-fat (using 2 pieces)*

BREAD/CEREAL

Whole wheat bread (using 4 slices)

Whole wheat 6" pita pockets (using 3)

Whole wheat wraps (using 3)

Whole wheat crackers, about 1½" square (using 48)

Rolled oats (using 1 cup)

Kashi 7 Whole Grain Puffs (using 3 cups)

Whole wheat pasta, any shape (using 2¼ cups cooked)

DRY GOODS

- Canola oil (using 1 tablespoon)
- Olive oil (4 tablespoons)
- Sunflower oil (using 3 tablespoons)
- Almonds (using 8 tablespoons)
- Brazil nuts, roasted or raw unsalted (using 6 tablespoons)
- Cannellini beans, no salt added (using 1¼ cups)
- Peanut butter (using 10 tablespoons)
- Green olives (using 40)
- Semisweet or dark chocolate chips (using ¾ cup)
- Cranberries, dried (using 8 tablespoons)
- Raisins (using 11 tablespoons)
- Roasted red peppers, jarred (using 4 tablespoons)
- Canola oil mayonnaise (using 2 teaspoons)
- Marinara sauce (using ½ cup)
- Chicken broth, reduced-sodium (using 2 cups)

MEAL REPLACEMENT BARS

- Luna: Chai Tea, Chocolate Pecan Pie, or Lemon Zest Bar or

Nature's Path: Optimum Energy Bar Blueberry Flax & Soy or Pomegran Cherry (using 3)

MEAT/SEAFOOD

- Chunk light water-pack tuna (using 6 ounces)

SPICES AND SEASONINGS

- Balsamic vinegar (using 4 tablespoons plus 2 teaspoons)
- Sherry vinegar (using 2 teaspoons)
- Hummus, 10-ounce container any flavor (using ½ cup)
- Pesto, 4-ounce container (using 2 tablespoons)
- Olive tapenade, 4.6-ounce container (You should be able to find this in the refrigerated section near the hummus or deli-style olives, or ask your store manager.) (using 4 tablespoons)

*We call for light or low-fat string cheese rather than part-skim because it is lower in saturated fat and calories. If you have trouble finding light or low-fat string cheese, though, feel free to substitute with part-skim string cheese.

DAY 15

BREAKFAST

Bar and Chocolate Chips: Have 1 Nature's Path Optimum Blueberry Flax & Soy or Pomegran Cherry bar (200) and 1/4 cup **semisweet or dark chocolate chips** (207).

Total calories: 407

LUNCH

Picnic Lunch: Spread 8 small whole wheat crackers (144) with 2 Laughing Cow Light Garlic & Herb Wedges (70). Have 10 large **green olives** (50), 1 cup baby carrots (50), and 1/4 cup hummus (100).

Total calories: 414

SNACK PACK

Crackers and Peanut Butter: Spread 8 small whole wheat crackers (144) with 2 tablespoons crunchy or smooth **peanut butter** (188) and top with 1 tablespoon raisins (33).

Total calories: 365

DINNER

White Bean Pasta: Mix 3/4 cup cooked whole wheat pasta, any shape (131), with 1 tablespoon **pesto sauce** (80), 2 teaspoons olive oil (79), 1/4 cup no-salt-added cannellini beans rinsed and drained (75), and 2 tablespoons roasted red peppers (6). Microwave to warm through.

Total calories: 377

DAY 16

Raisin and Nut Cereal: Mix 1½ cups Kashi 7 Whole Grain Puffs (105), 1 cup fat-free milk (80), 2 tablespoons **almonds** (109), and 2 tablespoons raisins (66).

Total calories: 360

LUNCH

Peanutty Cranberry Wrap: Spread 1 whole wheat wrap (140) with 2 tablespoons crunchy or smooth **peanut butter** (188) and 2 tablespoons dried cranberries (35). Have 1 cup baby carrots (50).

Total calories: 413

SNACK PACK

Deli Snack: Spread 8 small whole wheat crackers (144) with 2 tablespoons **black olive tapenade** (88). Serve with 1 cup baby carrots (50) and 3 ounces canned chunk light water-pack tuna (105) mixed with 1 teaspoon canola oil mayonnaise (33).

Total calories: 420

DINNER

Basil Bean Salad: Mix ¾ cup rinsed and drained cannellini beans (225), 1 small tomato, chopped (12), 1 tablespoon **olive oil** (119), 2 tablespoons balsamic vinegar (10), and ¼ teaspoon dried basil (0).

Total calories: 366

DAY 17

YOUR ULTIMATE 28-DAY EATING PLAN

BREAKFAST

Peach Almond Oatmeal: Cook ½ cup rolled oats with water to the consistency of your choice (150) and top with 2 tablespoons **almonds** (109) and 1 cup fresh or thawed frozen unsweetened sliced peaches (60). Have 1 cup fat-free milk (80).

Total calories: 399

LUNCH

Creamy Peanut Soup: Sauté ¼ cup chopped celery (4) and 2 tablespoons chopped onion (9) in 1 teaspoon olive oil (39) for 3 to 5 minutes or until soft. Add 1 cup reduced-sodium chicken broth (17), 1 teaspoon sherry vinegar (0), and 1 teaspoon lemon juice (1). Bring to a boil, then reduce heat and simmer for 5 to 7 minutes. Just before serving, stir in 2 tablespoons **peanut butter** (188). Mix ¼ cup fat-free ricotta cheese (50) and 1 tablespoon raisins (33); use as a dip for ½ whole wheat pita (70), toasted and cut into triangles.

Total calories: 410

SNACK PACK

Olive and Provolone Sandwich: Mix 10 **green olives,** sliced (50), with 1 minced garlic clove (5), 1 teaspoon balsamic vinegar (3), 1 teaspoon olive oil (39), and 1 teaspoon chopped fresh parsley (0). Let marinate overnight; fill 2 slices whole wheat bread (160) with the mixture and add 1 ounce reduced-fat provolone cheese (81). Serve with 1 medium orange, sliced (62).

Total calories: 400

DINNER

Veggie Pita: Fill 1 whole wheat pita (140) with a mixture of ½ cup baby spinach leaves (4), 1 cup mixed baby greens (9), ½ cup baby carrots, chopped (25), 1 tablespoon **sunflower oil** (120), 1 tablespoon balsamic vinegar (10), and 1 light or low-fat string cheese, chopped (60).

Total calories: 368

DAY 18

BREAKFAST

Bar and Chocolate Chips: Have 1 Nature's Path Optimum Blueberry Flax & Soy or Pomegran Cherry bar (200) and ¼ cup **semisweet or dark chocolate chips** (207).

Total calories: 407

LUNCH

Picnic Lunch: Spread 8 small whole wheat crackers (144) with 2 Laughing Cow Light Garlic & Herb Wedges (70). Have 10 large **green olives** (50), 1 cup baby carrots (50), and ¼ cup hummus (100).

Total calories: 414

SNACK PACK

Yogurt and Brazil Nuts: Top 6 ounces fat-free vanilla yogurt (155) with 2 tablespoons **Brazil nuts** (110) and 2 tablespoons raisins (66). Have 1 medium orange (62).

Total calories: 393

DINNER

Spinach Sunflower Stir-Fry: Heat 3 cups baby spinach leaves (24) in 1 tablespoon **sunflower oil** (120); add 1 medium orange, sectioned (62), and 2 tablespoons dried cranberries (45). Have 8 small whole wheat crackers (144).

Total calories: 395

YOUR ULTIMATE 28-DAY EATING PLAN

DAY 19

BREAKFAST

Raisin and Nut Cereal: Mix 1½ cups Kashi 7 Whole Grain Puffs (105), 1 cup fat-free milk (80), 2 tablespoons **almonds** (109), and 2 tablespoons raisins (66).

Total calories: 360

LUNCH

Cranberry Nut Ricotta Dip: Toast 1 whole wheat wrap (140) in a 200°F oven for 2 minutes, until crisp; break into pieces. Mix ½ cup fat-free ricotta cheese (100), 2 tablespoons dried cranberries (35), and 2 tablespoons **Brazil nuts,** chopped (110). Dip toasted pieces of wrap into ricotta mixture.

Total calories: 385

SNACK PACK

Olive and Provolone Sandwich: Mix 10 **green olives**, sliced (50), with 1 minced garlic clove (5), 1 teaspoon balsamic vinegar (3), 1 teaspoon olive oil (33), and 1 teaspoon chopped fresh parsley (0). Let marinate overnight; fill 2 slices whole wheat bread (160) with the mixture and add 1 ounce reduced-fat provolone cheese (81). Serve with 1 medium orange, sliced (62).

Total calories: 394

DINNER

White Bean Pasta: Mix ¾ cup cooked whole wheat pasta, any shape (131), with 1 tablespoon **pesto sauce** (80), 2 teaspoons olive oil (79), ¼ cup no-salt-added cannellini beans, rinsed and drained (75), and 2 tablespoons roasted red peppers (6). Microwave to warm through.

Total calories: 377

DAY 20

BREAKFAST

Peach Almond Oatmeal: Cook $\frac{1}{2}$ cup rolled oats with water to the consistency of your choice (150) and top with 2 tablespoons **almonds** (109) and 1 cup fresh or thawed frozen unsweetened sliced peaches (60). Have 1 cup fat-free milk (80).

Total calories: 399

LUNCH

Peanutty Cranberry Wrap: Spread 1 whole wheat wrap (140) with 2 tablespoons crunchy or smooth **peanut butter** (188) and 2 tablespoons dried cranberries (35). Have 1 cup baby carrots (50).

Total calories: 413

SNACK PACK

Yogurt and Brazil Nuts: Have 6 ounces fat-free vanilla yogurt (155) with 2 tablespoons **Brazil nuts** (110) and 2 tablespoons raisins (66). Have 1 medium orange (62).

Total calories: 393

DINNER

Cheesy Pasta with Spinach: Mix $\frac{3}{4}$ cup cooked whole wheat pasta, any shape (131), 1 tablespoon **canola oil** (124), 3 tablespoons shredded reduced-fat mozzarella cheese (52), 1 cup baby spinach leaves (8), and $\frac{1}{2}$ cup marinara sauce (60). Serve hot.

Total calories: 375

DAY 21

Bar and Chocolate Chips: Have 1 Nature's Path Optimum Blueberry Flax & Soy or Pomegran Cherry bar (200) and ¼ cup **semisweet or dark chocolate chips** (207).

Total calories: 407

LUNCH

Creamy Peanut Soup: Sauté ¼ cup chopped celery (4) and 2 tablespoons chopped onion (9) in 1 teaspoon olive oil (39) for 3 to 5 minutes or until soft. Add 1 cup reduced-sodium chicken broth (17), 1 teaspoon sherry vinegar (0), and 1 teaspoon lemon juice (1). Bring to a boil, then reduce heat and simmer for 5 to 7 minutes. Just before serving, stir in 2 tablespoons **peanut butter** (188). Mix ¼ cup fat-free ricotta cheese (50) and 1 tablespoon raisins (33); use as a dip for ½ whole wheat pita (70), toasted and cut into triangles.

Total calories: 410

SNACK

Deli Snack: Spread 8 small whole wheat crackers (144) with 2 tablespoons **black olive tapenade** (88). Serve with 1 cup baby carrots (50) and 3 ounces canned chunk light water-pack tuna (105) mixed with 1 teaspoon canola oil mayonnaise (33).

Total calories: 420

DINNER

Veggie Pita: Fill 1 whole wheat pita (140) with a mixture of ½ cup baby spinach leaves (4), 1 cup mixed baby greens (9), ½ cup baby carrots, chopped (25), 1 tablespoon **sunflower oil** (120), 1 tablespoon balsamic vinegar (10), and 1 light or low-fat string cheese, chopped (60).

Total calories: 368

DAY	MEAL	RECIPE	MUFA
22	Breakfast	Chocolate Raspberry Yogurt	Dark chocolate
22	Lunch	Roast Beef Pita	Black olives
22	Snack Pack	Cottage Cheese and Pineapple	Pecans
22	Dinner	Dijon Garden Burger Roll-Up	Pistachios
23	Breakfast	Bar and Hazelnuts	Hazelnuts
23	Lunch	Safflower Chicken Stir-Fry	Safflower oil
23	Snack Pack	Strawberry Chocolate Oatmeal	Dark chocolate
23	Dinner	Hearty Salad	Flaxseed oil
24	Breakfast	Pistachio Cereal	Pistachios
24	Lunch	Macadamia Pear Salad	Macadamia nuts
24	Snack Pack	Ginger Tahini Dip with Vegetables	Tahini
24	Dinner	Deli Wrap	Black olives
25	Breakfast	**Chocolate Raspberry Yogurt**	Dark chocolate
25	Lunch	Refried Bean Wrap	Flaxseed oil
25	Snack Pack	**Cottage Cheese and Pineapple**	Pecans
25	Dinner	Pistachio Herb Wrap	Pistachios
26	Breakfast	**Bar and Hazelnuts**	Hazelnuts
26	Lunch	**Roast Beef Pita**	Black olives
26	Snack Pack	**Ginger Tahini Dip with Vegetables**	Tahini
26	Dinner	**Hearty Salad**	Flaxseed oil
27	Breakfast	**Pistachio Cereal**	Pistachios
27	Lunch	**Safflower Chicken Stir-Fry**	Safflower oil
27	Snack Pack	**Strawberry Chocolate Oatmeal**	Dark chocolate
27	Dinner	**Deli Wrap**	Black olives
28	Breakfast	**Chocolate Raspberry Yogurt**	Dark chocolate
28	Lunch	**Macadamia Pear Salad**	Macadamia nuts
28	Snack Pack	**Cottage Cheese and Pineapple**	Pecans
28	Dinner	Roast Beef Wrap	Tahini

Bold = Repeated Recipe

SHOPPING LIST

Note: You'll notice some items listed in *italics*. If you've been following this plan exactly, you purchased these items in week 1 and should have enough of this food to fulfill what you need this week for the meal plan. We've added this information here just in case you're short on any ingredients for any reason.

PRODUCE

- Pears, 6 medium (using 6)
- Strawberries, 15 ounces fresh or 2 (10-ounce) packages frozen unsweetened (using 15 ounces)
- Raspberries, 15 ounces fresh or 2 (10-ounce) packages frozen unsweetened (using 15 ounces)
- Baby carrots, 12-ounce package (using 1 package)
- Baby greens, 10-ounce package mixed (using 1 package)
- Baby spinach leaves, 2 (9-ounce) packages (using 2 packages)
- Orange bell pepper, 1 medium (using 1)
- Tomatoes, 5 small (using 5)
- Onion, 1 medium (using 1)

- Cilantro, 1 bunch (optional) (using 1)

DAIRY

- Fat-free milk, ½ gallon (using 5 cups)
- Greek yogurt, 3 (6-ounce) containers fat-free (using 3 containers)
- Laughing Cow Light Garlic & Herb Wedges, 6-ounce package (using 6 wedges)
- Cottage cheese, 24-ounce container fat-free (using 3 cups)
- *String cheese, light or low-fat (using 2 pieces)**

FROZEN FOODS

- *Meatless chicken-style nuggets (using 8)*
- *Veggie burgers (using 1)*

BREAD/CEREAL

- *Whole wheat 6" pita pockets (using 4)*
- Whole wheat wraps, 8" diameter, 1 (6-count) package (using 4)
- *Rolled oats (using 1 cup)*
- *Kashi 7 Whole Grain Puffs (using 4 cups)*

DRY GOODS

☐ Flaxseed oil, cold-pressed (using 3 tablespoons)

☐ Safflower oil (using 2 tablespoons)

☐ Sesame oil (using 6 teaspoons)

☐ Hazelnuts (using 4 tablespoons)

☐ Macadamia nuts, raw unsalted (using 4 tablespoons)

☐ Pecans, roasted or raw unsalted (using 6 tablespoons)

☐ Pistachios, raw unsalted (using 8 tablespoons)

☐ Kidney beans (using 1/3 cup)

☐ Black olives, large (using 50)

☐ Semisweet or dark chocolate chips (using 1 1/4 cups)

☐ Pineapple tidbits packed in juice, canned (using 24 ounces)

☐ Raisins (using 8 tablespoons)

☐ Dijon mustard (using 2 teaspoons)

☐ Canola oil mayonnaise (using 5 teaspoons)

☐ Agave nectar (using 5 teaspoons)

MEAL REPLACEMENT BARS

☐ Luna: Chai Tea, Chocolate Pecan Pie, or Lemon Zest Bar or

Nature's Path: Optimum Energy Bar Blueberry Flax & Soy or Pomegran Cherry (using 2)

MEAT/SEAFOOD

☐ Organic deli roast beef, 2 (6-ounce) packages (using 11 ounces)**

☐ Organic deli turkey breast, 8-ounce package (using 8 ounces)**

SPICES AND SEASONINGS

☐ Balsamic vinegar (using 2 tablespoons)

☐ Rice vinegar (using 3 tablespoons plus 1 teaspoon)

☐ Ground ginger (using 1/2 teaspoon)

☐ Hummus, 8-ounce package (using 1/2 cup)

☐ Tahini, 4-ounce package (using 6 tablespoons)

*We call for light or low-fat string cheese rather than part-skim because it is lower in saturated fat and calories. If you have trouble finding light or low-fat string cheese, though, feel free to substitute with part-skim string cheese.

**We call for organic deli meat because it is generally lower in sodium and fat. If you choose to purchase nonorganic meat, please look for low-sodium choices.

DAY 22

BREAKFAST

Chocolate Raspberry Yogurt: Mix 6 ounces fat-free Greek yogurt (80) with 1/4 cup **semisweet or dark chocolate chips** (207) and 1 cup fresh or thawed frozen unsweetened raspberries (70). Drizzle with 1 teaspoon agave nectar (20).

Total calories: 377

LUNCH

Roast Beef Pita: Spread 1 whole wheat pita (140) with 2 teaspoons canola oil mayonnaise (66) and fill with 10 sliced **black olives** (50) and 4 ounces organic deli roast beef (129).

Total calories: 385

SNACK PACK

Cottage Cheese and Pineapple: Mix 1 cup fat-free cottage cheese (180), 8 ounces pineapple tidbits canned in juice, drained (120), and 2 tablespoons **pecans** (90).

Total calories: 390

DINNER

Dijon Garden Burger Roll-Up: Fill 1 whole wheat wrap (140) with 1 cooked and crumbled veggie burger (100) dressed with 2 teaspoons Dijon mustard (10) and 1 teaspoon canola oil mayonnaise (33), 1/2 cup baby spinach leaves (4), 1 small tomato, diced (12), and 2 tablespoons **pistachios** (88).

Total calories: 387

DAY 23

BREAKFAST

Bar and Hazelnuts: Have 1 Luna Chai Tea, Chocolate Pecan Pie, or Lemon Zest bar (180) with 2 tablespoons **hazelnuts** (110), 1 tablespoon raisins (33), and 1 cup fat-free milk (80).

Total calories: 403

LUNCH

Safflower Chicken Stir-Fry: Sauté ¼ cup diced onion (16) and ½ cup chopped baby carrots (25) in 1 tablespoon **high-oleic safflower oil** (120) until onions are translucent, about 4 to 5 minutes. Heat 4 meatless chicken-style nuggets (172) according to the package directions; add to the pan with 3 cups baby spinach leaves (24) and stir until spinach is wilted, about 1 minute.

Total calories: 357

SNACK PACK

Strawberry Chocolate Oatmeal: Cook ½ cup rolled oats with water to the consistency of your choice (150); stir in 1 cup fresh or thawed frozen unsweetened strawberries (52) and ¼ cup **semisweet or dark chocolate chips** (207).

Total calories: 409

DINNER

Hearty Salad: Mix 3 cups baby greens (27), 1 small tomato, diced (12), ½ cup baby carrots, chopped (25), 1 light or low-fat string cheese, chopped (60), and 5 large black olives, chopped (25). Drizzle with 1 tablespoon cold-pressed organic **flaxseed oil** (120) and 1 tablespoon balsamic vinegar (5). Serve with a toasted whole wheat pita (140).

Total calories: 414

DAY 24

BREAKFAST

Pistachio Cereal: Mix 2 cups Kashi 7 Whole Grain Puffs (140), 1 cup fat-free milk (80), 2 tablespoons **pistachios** (88), and 2 tablespoons raisins (66).

Total calories: 374

LUNCH

Macadamia Pear Salad: Mix 3 cups baby spinach leaves (24), 1 medium pear, sliced (103), 1 tablespoon raisins (33), 1 small tomato, diced (12), 2 teaspoons sesame oil (80), 1 tablespoon rice vinegar (0), and 2 tablespoons **macadamia nuts** (120).

Total calories: 372

SNACK PACK

Ginger Tahini Dip with Vegetables: Combine 2 tablespoons **tahini** (178) with 1 teaspoon chopped fresh cilantro (0), 1 teaspoon toasted sesame oil (33), 1 teaspoon agave nectar (20), and ¼ teaspoon ground ginger (0) as dip for ½ cup sliced orange bell peppers (23). Have with 1 medium pear (103), sliced and spread with 2 Laughing Cow Garlic & Herb Wedges (70).

Total calories: 426

DINNER

Deli Wrap: Spread 4 ounces organic deli turkey breast (131) with ¼ cup hummus (100), sprinkle with 10 sliced **black olives** (50), and roll up. Have 1 medium pear (103).

Total calories: 384

DAY 25

BREAKFAST

Chocolate Raspberry Yogurt: Mix 6 ounces fat-free Greek yogurt (80) with 1/4 cup **semisweet or dark chocolate chips** (207) and 1 cup fresh or thawed frozen unsweetened raspberries (70). Drizzle with 1 teaspoon agave nectar (20).

Total calories: 377

LUNCH

Refried Bean Wrap: Warm 1/4 cup diced onion (16), 1 tablespoon balsamic vinegar (5), and 1 tablespoon cold-pressed organic **flaxseed oil** (120) in a skillet. Stir in 1/3 cup mashed no-salt-added kidney beans (100). Spread on 1 whole wheat wrap (140).

Total calories: 381

SNACK PACK

Cottage Cheese and Pineapple: Mix 1 cup fat-free cottage cheese (180), 8 ounces pineapple tidbits canned in juice, drained (120), and 2 tablespoons **pecans** (90).

Total calories: 390

DINNER

Pistachio Herb Wrap: Spread 1 whole wheat wrap (140) with 2 Laughing Cow Garlic & Herb Wedges (70) and sprinkle with 2 tablespoons **pistachios** (88). Have 1 cup fat-free milk (80).

Total calories: 378

DAY 26

BREAKFAST

Bar and Hazelnuts: Have 1 Luna Chai Tea, Chocolate Pecan Pie, or Lemon Zest bar (180) with 2 tablespoons **hazelnuts** (110), 1 tablespoon raisins (33), and 1 cup fat-free milk (80).

Total calories: 403

LUNCH

Roast Beef Pita: Spread 1 whole wheat pita (140) with 2 teaspoons canola oil mayonnaise (66) and fill with 10 sliced **black olives** (50) and 4 ounces organic deli roast beef (129).

Total calories: 385

SNACK PACK

Ginger Tahini Dip with Vegetables: Combine 2 tablespoons **tahini** (178) with 1 teaspoon chopped fresh cilantro (0), 1 teaspoon toasted sesame oil (33), 1 teaspoon agave nectar (20), and $1/4$ teaspoon ground ginger (0) as a dip for $1/2$ cup sliced orange bell peppers (23). Have 1 medium pear (103), sliced and spread with 2 Laughing Cow Garlic & Herb Wedges (70).

Total calories: 426

DINNER

Hearty Salad: Mix 3 cups baby greens (27), 1 small tomato, diced (12), $1/2$ cup baby carrots, chopped (25), 1 light or low-fat string cheese, chopped (60), and 5 large black olives, chopped (25). Drizzle with 1 tablespoon cold-pressed organic **flaxseed oil** (120) and 1 tablespoon balsamic vinegar (5). Serve with a toasted whole wheat pita (140).

Total calories: 414

DAY 27

BREAKFAST

Pistachio Cereal: Mix 2 cups Kashi 7 Whole Grain Puffs (140), 1 cup fat-free milk (80), 2 tablespoons **pistachios** (88), and 2 tablespoons raisins (66).

Total calories: 374

LUNCH

Safflower Chicken Stir-Fry: Sauté ¼ cup diced onion (16) and ½ cup chopped baby carrots (25) in 1 tablespoon **high-oleic safflower oil** (120) until onions are translucent, about 4 to 5 minutes. Heat 4 meatless chicken-style nuggets (172) according to the package directions; add to the pan with 3 cups baby spinach leaves (24) and stir until spinach is wilted, about 1 minute.

Total calories: 357

SNACK PACK

Strawberry Chocolate Oatmeal: Cook ½ cup rolled oats with water to the consistency of your choice (150); stir in 1 cup fresh or thawed frozen unsweetened strawberries (52) and ¼ cup **semisweet or dark chocolate chips** (207).

Total calories: 409

DINNER

Deli Wrap: Spread 4 ounces organic deli turkey breast (131) with ¼ cup hummus (100), sprinkle with 10 sliced **black olives** (50), and roll up. Have 1 medium pear (103).

Total calories: 384

DAY 28

Chocolate Raspberry Yogurt: Mix 6 ounces fat-free Greek yogurt (80) with $1/4$ cup **semisweet or dark chocolate chips** (207) and 1 cup fresh or thawed frozen unsweetened raspberries (70). Drizzle with 1 teaspoon agave nectar (20).

Total calories: 377

Macadamia Pear Salad: Mix 3 cups baby spinach leaves (24), 1 medium pear, sliced (103), 1 tablespoon raisins (33), 1 small tomato, diced (12), 2 teaspoons sesame oil (80), 1 tablespoon rice vinegar (0), and 2 tablespoons **macadamia nuts** (120).

Total calories: 372

Cottage Cheese and Pineapple: Mix 1 cup fat-free cottage cheese (180), 8 ounces pineapple tidbits canned in juice, drained (120), and 2 tablespoons **pecans** (90).

Total calories: 390

Roast Beef Wrap: Spread 1 whole wheat wrap (140) with 2 tablespoons **tahini** (178); fill with 3 ounces organic deli roast beef (97) and $1/2$ cup baby spinach leaves (4).

Total calories: 419

6.

ADDITIONAL
QUICK-AND-EASY
MEALS &
SNACK PACKS

When you need some variation from Your Ultimate 28-Day Eating
Plan, look no further than these Quick-and-Easy Meals and Snack
Packs. You can substitute any of these for any meal on the diet. They're
all simple, throw-together options with minimal ingredients, yet they're
tasty and healthy. What a great combination!

BREAKFASTS

Tomato Basil Ricotta Wrap:
Fill 1 whole wheat wrap (140) with a mixture of 1 small tomato, chopped (12), 1 teaspoon chopped fresh or $\frac{1}{3}$ teaspoon dried basil (0), $\frac{1}{2}$ cup fat-free ricotta cheese (100), and 1 tablespoon **olive oil** (119).

■ Total calories: 371

Raisin Almond Wrap: Spread 1 whole wheat wrap (140) with 2 tablespoons **almond butter** (200) and sprinkle with 2 tablespoons raisins (66).

■ Total calories: 406

Peanut Butter Toast and Strawberries: Spread 2 slices toasted whole wheat bread (160) with 2 tablespoons crunchy or smooth **peanut butter** (188). Serve with 1 cup sliced fresh or thawed frozen unsweetened strawberries (52).

■ Total calories: 400

Pumpkin Raisin Wrap: Mix $\frac{1}{2}$ cup fat-free cottage cheese (90) with $\frac{1}{4}$ teaspoon ground cinnamon (0), 1 tablespoon raisins (33), and 2 tablespoons pumpkin seeds (148). Fill 1 whole wheat wrap (140) with the mixture.

■ Total calories: 411

Apple Cobbler: Mix $1\frac{1}{2}$ cups Kashi 7 Whole Grain Puffs (105), with 1 medium apple, chopped (95), 2 tablespoons **walnuts** (82), and 1 cup fat-free milk (80). Heat in the microwave on high for 1 minute or until warm. Sprinkle with $\frac{1}{4}$ teaspoon each of ground cinnamon (0) and ground nutmeg (0).

■ Total calories: 362

LUNCHES

Cheesy Roast Beef Muffin:
Spread 1 toasted whole wheat English muffin (140) with 1 Laughing Cow Light Garlic & Herb Wedge (35) and 2 tablespoons **cashews** (148). Fill with 2 ounces organic deli roast beef (65).

■ Total calories: 388

Spiced Edamame: Mix 1 cup shelled and boiled **edamame** (298) with $\frac{1}{4}$ teaspoon ground cumin (0) and 1 shake of cayenne pepper (0). Serve with $\frac{1}{2}$ cup cooked brown rice (109).

■ Total calories: 407

Grapefruit Walnut Salad: Mix 3 cups shredded romaine lettuce (24), 2 tablespoons **walnuts** (82), 1 grapefruit, sectioned (120), and $\frac{1}{2}$ teaspoon ground black pepper (0). Serve with 2 slices toasted whole wheat bread (160) spread with 2 tablespoons mashed Hass avocado (48).

■ Total calories: 434

Walnut Raisin Pita: Fill 1 whole wheat pita (140) with a mixture of 2 tablespoons **walnuts** (82), 1 tablespoon raisins (33), 3 ounces organic deli chicken breast (75), 1 small tomato, diced (12), $\frac{1}{2}$ cup shredded romaine lettuce (4), and 1 teaspoon olive oil (39).

■ Total calories: 385

Monterey Corn Tortilla: Sprinkle 3 small corn tortillas (171) with 4 tablespoons shredded Monterey Jack cheese (81); heat under the broiler or in the toaster oven to warm. Top with $\frac{1}{4}$ cup salsa (18), $\frac{1}{4}$ cup sliced **Hass avocado** (96), and 1 cup baby spinach leaves (8).

■ Total calories: 374

Mexican Pita: Fill 1 whole wheat pita (140) with a mixture of $\frac{1}{4}$ cup rinsed and drained kidney beans (75), 2 tablespoons salsa (9), 1 tablespoon **olive oil** (119), $\frac{1}{2}$ cup shredded romaine lettuce (4), and 2 tablespoons shredded reduced-fat Cheddar cheese (40).

■ Total calories: 387

Peanut Mango Chutney Roll: Spread 1 whole wheat soft tortilla (140) with 1 teaspoon peanut butter (31). Top with 2 tablespoons **peanuts** (110), 2 ounces organic deli chicken breast (50), and $\frac{1}{2}$ cup fresh or frozen mango chunks (60) sprinkled with 1 teaspoon lime juice (1).

■ Total calories: 392

Speedy Chicken Satay: Fill 1 whole wheat soft tortilla (140) with a mixture of 4 ounces organic deli chicken breast (100), 2 tablespoons **peanuts** (110), 1 teaspoon chopped fresh tarragon (0), and 2 tablespoons fat-free plain yogurt (15).

■ Total calories: 365

Pecan Cilantro Turkey: Sauté 4 ounces raw ground turkey breast (120) in 2 teaspoons olive oil (78) until cooked. Stir in $1/4$ cup cooked brown rice (55), 2 tablespoons **pecans** (90), 1 teaspoon chopped cilantro (0), $1/2$ teaspoon chipotle chile pepper (0), and $1/4$ teaspoon ground black pepper (0). Heat through. Have $1/2$ cup red or green grapes (52).

■ Total calories: 395

Cranberry Pistachio Pita: Fill 1 whole wheat pita (140) with a mixture of $1/2$ cup fat-free ricotta cheese (90), 1 teaspoon agave nectar (20), 2 tablespoons dried cranberries (45), and 2 tablespoons **pistachios** (88).

■ Total calories: 383

Salmon and Brown Rice: Mix 4 ounces canned wild salmon (180), 2 teaspoons olive oil (78), 2 tablespoons **walnuts** (82), and $1/3$ cup cooked brown rice (73).

■ Total calories: 413

Turkey Roll-Up: Spread 1 whole wheat tortilla (140) with 1 tablespoon canola oil mayonnaise (99) and fill with 3 ounces organic deli turkey breast (75), 2 tablespoons **walnuts** (82), 1 teaspoon raisins (11), and $1/2$ cup shredded romaine lettuce (4).

■ Total calories: 411

Bean and Rice Salad: Top $1/2$ cup cooked brown rice (109) with a mixture of $1/3$ cup rinsed and drained pinto beans (83), $1/4$ cup chopped **Hass avocado** (96), 1 small tomato, diced (12), 2 teaspoons olive oil (78), 2 tablespoons salsa (9), 2 tablespoons lime juice (6), and a shake of black pepper (0).

■ Total calories: 393

California Pita: Fill 1 whole wheat pita (140) with 4 ounces organic deli turkey (100), 1 small tomato, diced (12), $1/4$ cup chopped **Hass avocado** (96), and $1/2$ cup baby spinach leaves (4).

■ Total calories: 352

Chicken, Cheese, and Olive Wrap: Fill 1 whole wheat soft wrap (140) with 4 tablespoons shredded reduced-fat Monterey Jack cheese (81), 10 large **black olives,** sliced (50), and 4 ounces organic deli chicken breast (100).

■ Total calories: 371

Waffle with Almond Butter Spread: Top 1 toasted frozen whole grain waffle (100) with 2 tablespoons **almond butter** (200) blended with 2 tablespoons fat-free plain yogurt (15). Top with 1 cup sliced fresh or thawed frozen unsweetened strawberries (52).

■ Total calories: 367

Edamame Salad: Mix together 1 cup shelled and boiled **edamame** (298), 1 tablespoon lemon juice (4), 1 teaspoon olive oil (33), 1/2 cup cooked corn (66), and 1/4 cup diced red bell pepper (12).

■ Total calories: 413

Bar and Pecans: Have 1 Luna Chai Tea, Chocolate Pecan Pie, or Lemon Zest bar (180) with 2 tablespoons **pecans** (90), 4 ounces pineapple tidbits canned in juice (60), and 4 small whole wheat crackers (72).

■ Total calories: 402

Tropical Cottage Cheese: Have 1 cup fat-free cottage cheese (180), 2 tablespoons **sunflower seeds** (90), 4 ounces pineapple tidbits canned in juice (60), and 4 small whole wheat crackers (72).

■ Total calories: 402

Mediterranean Bean Roll-Ups: Warm 2 small corn tortillas (114) and spread with a mixture of 1/2 cup rinsed and drained cannellini beans (150), 1 tablespoon balsamic vinegar (5), 1 teaspoon olive oil (39), 1 teaspoon chopped fresh basil (0), and a shake of chili powder (0). Top with 1/4 cup sliced **Hass avocado** (96) and 1/2 cup shredded romaine lettuce (4).

■ Total calories: 408

Mini Pizzas: Spread 3 small corn tortillas (171) with 1/2 cup marinara sauce (60), 10 large **black olives**, sliced (50), 1/4 cup shredded reduced-fat Cheddar cheese (80), and 1/2 cup thinly sliced red bell pepper (24). Place under the broiler or in a toaster oven until the cheese begins to melt.

■ Total calories: 385

Monterey Jack Pita Triangles:
Slice 1 whole wheat pita into quarters (140) and top with 2 tablespoons salsa (9), $\frac{1}{4}$ cup chopped red bell pepper (12), $\frac{1}{4}$ cup chopped yellow bell pepper (12), 4 tablespoons shredded reduced-fat Monterey Jack cheese (81), and 10 large **black olives,** sliced (50). Place under the broiler or in a toaster oven to warm. Have with 1 medium apple (95).

■ Total calories: 399

Olive and Mozzarella Sandwich: Sprinkle 2 slices whole wheat bread (160) with 10 large **black olives,** sliced (50), and $\frac{1}{4}$ cup shredded reduced-fat mozzarella cheese (70). Place under the broiler or in a toaster oven to warm, if desired. Have with 1 medium pear (103).

■ Total calories: 383

Chocolate Strawberry Yogurt:
Mix 8 ounces fat-free plain yogurt (120) with $\frac{1}{4}$ cup **semisweet chocolate chips** (207) and 1 cup sliced fresh or thawed frozen unsweetened strawberries (52).

■ Total calories: 379

Sweet Surprise Cereal: Melt $\frac{1}{4}$ cup **semisweet chocolate chips** in a medium bowl in the microwave for 40 to 50 seconds (207). Add $1\frac{1}{2}$ cups Kashi 7 Whole Grain Puffs (105) and 2 tablespoons raisins (66); stir to blend and allow to cool before eating.

■ Total calories: 378

7.

WHEN YOU'RE
OUT AND
ABOUT

The Quick-and-Easy Meals and Snack Packs in this plan make it easy for you to follow the *Flat Belly Diet* rules when you have the time to plan ahead and make your meals. But what about those times when you're traveling, out running errands, or stuck in the office and you forgot to bring your *Flat Belly Diet* meals? Look no further than this chapter to help you select the best choices to stick to your diet when you're out and about.

In this chapter, you'll find recommendations for specific brand-name products, which *Prevention* magazine has screened to make sure they're free of trans fats and artificial sweeteners and which can provide a great shortcut for meals and snacks when you're short on time (see *Flat Belly Diet*–Friendly Products, opposite). You'll also find lists of *Flat Belly Diet*–friendly entrées on the menus of popular national restaurant and fast-food chains, so that you can still enjoy dinners out with your family and friends without sabotaging your weight loss (see Restaurant Rescue, page 113). Finally, you'll find advice on making the best food choices whenever you're stuck at the airport, in front of a vending machine, or in other spots where healthy eating may be a challenge (see Best Meal Choices, page 123).

CAN A HOTEL BREAKFAST BE *FLAT BELLY DIET* FRIENDLY?

Over the past year, I've done a lot of traveling, and that means a lot of "continental breakfasts." Someone should start calling these "Croissant Breakfasts" because these buttery pastries seem to be the tastiest things available. I've learned that eating healthy in hotels involves a lot of preparing ahead. To make your own *Flat Belly Diet* breakfast, pack small boxes of cereal, whole wheat crackers, or packets of plain instant oatmeal as well as nuts or seeds (premeasured in MUFA-size portions in individual zip-top bags), fruit packed in juice or water in individual serving cups, and individual portions of shelf-stable milk, whether plain fat-free soy, almond, enriched rice, or dairy milk.

FLAT BELLY DIET–FRIENDLY PRODUCTS

It's extremely important that you understand that none of the manufacturers of the products mentioned here have paid to be included in this book. Instead, these brands have been thoroughly reviewed, tested, and selected based on their ingredients, nutritional value, taste, and quality. They're suggestions only. If you can't find them, no worries. Feel free to choose the brands that are easily available to you and that fit your budget and location. Just keep in mind the MUFA Meal Maker Guidelines:

- ○ Guideline #1: Consume no more than 4 grams of saturated fat per meal.

- ○ Guideline #2: Ban trans fat.

- ○ Guideline #3: Avoid artificial sweeteners, flavorings, and preservatives.

- ○ Guideline #4: Limit sodium to less than 2,300 milligrams a day.

As always, choose products with ingredients you can easily recognize and pronounce and foods (including frozen meals) that are made with whole grains, real produce, lean protein, and low-fat dairy.

PREPARED MUFA-RICH FOODS

	MUFA	BRAND/PRODUCT
OILS	Olive Oil	● 365 Organic Everyday Value (Whole Foods) Extra Virgin Olive Oil ● Bertolli Extra Virgin Olive Oil ● Goya Extra Virgin Olive Oil ● Trader Joe's Extra Virgin Olive Oil
	Pesto	● Buitoni Pesto with Basil ● Classico Sun-Dried Tomato Pesto
NUTS, LEGUMES, AND SEEDS	Almond Butter	● Earth Balance Natural Almond Butter ● Futters Nut Butters All Natural Almond Butter
	Cashew Butter	● Once Again Organic Cashew Nut Butter ● Futters Nut Butters All Natural Cashew Butter
	Peanut Butter	● Smart Balance ● Smucker's Natural or Smucker's Organic
	Sunflower Seed Butter	● SunButter Natural ● SunGold Natural
	Tahini	● Sabra Tahini Spread & Dip
AVOCADOS	Guacamole	● AvoClassic Guacamole ● Wholly Guacamole
OLIVES	Olive Tapenade	● Cantaré Olive Tapenade ● Mt. Vikos Kalamata Olive Spread
DARK CHOCOLATE	Dark or Semisweet Chocolate	● Chocolove Organic Dark Cocoa ● Dagoba Organic Sweet Dark Chocolate Bar ● Sunspire Organic Semi-Sweet Chocolate Chips ● Trader Joe's Organic Dark Chocolate 73% Super Dark Bar ● Woodstock Farms Organic Chips, Dark Chocolate Confections

MEAL BUILDING BLOCKS

FOOD	BRAND/PRODUCT
Deli Meat Slices	● Applegate Farms Antibiotic-Free deli meats: roasted, herb, smoked, and honey & maple turkey slices; natural roast beef slices; natural ham slices; uncured black forest ham ● Coleman Natural: honey and oven roasted turkey; medium-rare roast beef; Virginia brand, uncured, and quarter ham slices ● Hormel all-natural deli sandwich meats: oven roasted, smoked, and honey turkey; honey, smoked, and cooked ham; roast beef slices
Tuna	● Bumble Bee Chunk Light Tuna in Water
Salmon	● Bumble Bee Wild Pink Salmon
Egg Whites	● All-Whites 100% Liquid Egg Whites ● Better'n Eggs Liquid Egg Whites ● Egg Beaters Whites ● Organic Valley Egg Whites
Meat Substitutes	● Lightlife: Smart ground original crumbles; Smart taco and burrito crumbles; turkey, ham, and bologna Smart Deli slices; Smart Deli pepperoni; light burgers ● Yves Meatless: turkey, ham, smoked chicken, and roast beef deli slices; meatless ground round original; meatless ground turkey; meatless beef burger; meatless chicken burger
Meatless Chicken-Style Nuggets	● Health Is Wealth Chicken-Free Nuggets ● Trader Joe's Soy Nuggets or Meatless Chicken-Style Nuggets
Veggie Burgers	● Amy's Kitchen American Veggie Burgers (120 calories) ● Boca Original Vegan veggie burgers ● Dr. Praeger's: California Veggie Burgers, Tex Mex Veggie Burgers ● Gardenburger: Portabella, Flame Grilled, Veggie Medley, The Original, Black Bean Chipotle ● Morning Star Farms: Grillers Prime Veggie Burgers, Grillers Original, Grillers Vegan Veggie Burgers

LEAN PROTEIN

FOOD	BRAND/PRODUCT
DAIRY AND DAIRY ALTERNATIVES	
Cheese	• Horizon Organic part-skim mozzarella string cheese • Laughing Cow cheese wedges: Light Garlic & Herb, Original Creamy Swiss • Organic Valley part-skim mozzarella sticks • Polly-O String Cheese—mozzarella, made with 2% milk, natural, reduced fat • Sargento light string cheese
Fat-Free Milk	• Horizon Organic fat-free milk • Trader Joe's organic or regular fat-free milk
Soy Milk	• Silk unsweetened plain soy milk, light vanilla soy milk • WestSoy organic unsweetened plain soy milk, unsweetened chocolate soy milk, unsweetened vanilla soy milk
Yogurt	• Dannon All Natural: fat-free plain yogurt (80 calories per 6 oz) • Dannon All Natural: low-fat flavored yogurt (150 calories per 6 oz) • Stonyfield Farm Fat Free flavored yogurts: all flavors (130 calories per 6 oz) • Stonyfield Farm Fat Free plain yogurt (80 to 90 calories per 6 oz)
FRUITS AND VEGETABLES	
Frozen Fruits	• Cascadian Farm organic blueberries, strawberries, blackberries, cherries, sliced peaches, harvest berries • Dole unsweetened or no-sugar-added frozen fruits: blueberries, strawberries, blackberries, cherries, sliced peaches, pineapple chunks, mango

FOOD	BRAND/PRODUCT
Breads *(about 80 calories per slice/2 to 3 grams of fiber per serving)*	<ul><li>Pepperidge Farm 100% Whole Wheat bread</li><li>Thomas' 100% Whole Wheat English Muffins and multigrain pitas</li><li>Thomas' Sahara Pitas: mini and regular size (multi-grain and original) and Wraps (Wheat and White)</li><li>Food For Life Ezekiel 4:9 Organic Sprouted Bread: Regular or Cinnamon Raisin</li></ul>
Cereal	<ul><li>Arrowhead Mills: puffed rice, puffed wheat, millet</li><li>Barbara's Bakery: Puffins Honey Rice, Original, Cinnamon</li><li>Cream of Wheat</li><li>Erewhon: Corn Flakes, Crispy Brown Rice, Rice Twice</li><li>Health Valley: Organic Blue Corn Flakes</li><li>Kashi 7 Whole Grain Puffs</li><li>Nature's Path: Organic multigrain flakes, corn flakes, Flax plus flakes, Synergy 8 whole grains</li></ul>
Crackers	<ul><li>Health Valley Organic: Stoned Wheat, Whole Wheat, Sesame, Garden Herb, Cracked Pepper</li><li>Kashi TLC Crackers: Fire Roasted Vegetable, Honey Sesame, Original 7 Grain (use 7 crackers as a serving size)</li><li>Pepperidge Farm Harvest Wheat Crackers, Wheat Crisps</li><li>Ryvita Crispbread Crackers: Dark Rye, Sesame Rye</li><li>Wasa Crispbread: Multi Grain, Oats, Light Rye, Sesame Toast, Crisp'n Light 7 Grain, Fiber Rye, Sourdough Rye</li></ul>
Frozen Waffles	<ul><li>Kashi GoLean Strawberry Flax, Blueberry, or Original</li><li>Nature's Path Organic Flax Plus Waffles</li><li>Van's: 97% fat-free, original</li></ul>

FOOD	BRAND/PRODUCT
SEASONINGS AND CONDIMENTS	
Pasta Sauce	● Barilla Pasta Sauce: Marinara, Mushroom & Garlic, Roasted Garlic ● Contadina Buitoni Marinara Sauce ● Newman's Own Sauce: Marinara Sauce, Marinara with Mushrooms Sauce, Sockarooni Sauce, Roasted Garlic & Peppers Sauce, Fire Roasted Tomato & Garlic Sauce
Salad Dressing	● Annie's Naturals: Goddess Dressing, Organic Green Goddess Dressing, Organic Asian Sesame Dressing ● Newman's Own Lighten Up: Balsamic Vinaigrette, Roast Garlic Balsamic, Low-Fat Sesame Ginger, Sun Dried Tomato
COMPLETE MEALS	
Frozen Dinners	● Amy's Kitchen Chili & Cornbread Whole Meal, Black Bean Enchilada Whole Meal, Indian Mattar Paneer, Indian Vegetable Korma, Organic Brown Rice and Vegetables Bowl, Brown Rice, Black Eyed Peas, & Veggies Bowl, Teriyaki Bowl, Veggie Loaf Whole Meal, Indian Mattar Tofu, Light in Sodium Shepherd's Pie ● Boca Meatless Chili ● Cedarlane Low-Fat Pizza Veggie Wrap ● Gardenburger Wraps (240 calories): Black Bean Chipotle Wrap, Margherita Pizza Wrap ● Kashi Lemon Rosemary Chicken, Southwest Style Chicken ● Kashi Lime Cilantro Shrimp, Sweet & Sour Chicken, Black Bean Mango, Lemon Rosemary Chicken, Chicken Pasta Pomodoro, Southwest Style Chicken ● Seeds of Change (300 to 320 calories): Hanalei Vegetarian Chicken Teriyaki, Lasagna Calabrese with Eggplant and Portabello Mushrooms, Spicy Thai Peanut Noodles ● Yves Meatless Penne
Meal Replacement Bars	● Clif Bars: any flavor ● Kashi TLC Chewy Granola Bars and Crunchy Granola Bars: any flavor ● Larabar: any flavor ● Luna Bars: any flavor ● Nature's Path Optimum energy bars: any flavor ● Odwalla bars: any flavor

MAKE IT A *FLAT BELLY DIET* MEAL

When you're really pressed for time but are craving a hot meal, you can add a MUFA to one of the following frozen dinners to make them a *Flat Belly Diet* meal. You can add any MUFA you choose, as long as it fits in the 400-calorie range, but here are some suggestions.

Amy's Kitchen Chili & Cornbread Whole Meal (340) with 10 large **green or black olives** (50)
TOTAL CALORIES: 390

Amy's Kitchen Black Bean Vegetable Enchilada—have both servings (360) with 10 large **green or black olives** (50)
TOTAL CALORIES: 410

Amy's Kitchen Indian Mattar Paneer (320) with 2 tablespoons **walnuts** (82)
TOTAL CALORIES: 402

Amy's Kitchen Indian Vegetable Korma (310) with 2 tablespoons **walnuts** (82)
TOTAL CALORIES: 392

Amy's Kitchen Organic Brown Rice, Black-Eyed Peas, & Veggies Bowl (290) with 2 tablespoons **peanuts** (110)
TOTAL CALORIES: 400

Amy's Kitchen Teriyaki Bowl (290) with 2 tablespoons **peanuts** (110)
TOTAL CALORIES: 400

Amy's Kitchen Veggie Loaf Whole Meal (290) with 2 tablespoons **peanuts** (110)
TOTAL CALORIES: 400

Amy's Kitchen Indian Mattar Tofu (260) with 2 tablespoons **pumpkin seeds** (148)
TOTAL CALORIES: 408

Amy's Kitchen Light in Sodium Shepherd's Pie (160) with 1 medium piece fruit (60) and 2 tablespoons **pumpkin seeds** (148)
TOTAL CALORIES: 368

Kashi Lemon Rosemary Chicken (330) with 10 large **green or black olives** (50)
TOTAL CALORIES: 380

Kashi Southwest Style Chicken (240) with 2 tablespoons **pumpkin seeds** (148)
TOTAL CALORIES: 388

Seeds of Change Spicy Thai Peanut Noodles (350) with 10 large **green or black olives** (50)
TOTAL CALORIES: 400

Seeds of Change Hanalei Vegetarian Chicken Teriyaki (300) with 2 tablespoons **peanuts** (110)
TOTAL CALORIES: 410

SPECIAL DIETS

Here are some recommended brands to include if you have any special dietary needs.

Gluten Free
Deli slices: Applegate Farms Turkey
Dried plums: Sunsweet Ones
Puffed rice cereal: Arrowhead Mills, Erewhon
Unsweetened corn flakes: Health Valley, Nature's Path

Dairy Free
Deli slices: Applegate Farms Turkey
Milk alternatives: Almond Breeze Almond Milk
Soy cheese: Tofutti, Veggie Slices
Snack alternative: Luna Bars

Soy Free
Meat and veggie burgers: Applegate Farms, Amy's Kitchen California Veggie Burger, Gardenburger GardenVegan Burger
Cheese: Galaxy Nutritional Foods Rice Cheese Slices, Horizon Organic Cheddar Slices
Fat-free milk: Horizon Organic, Organic Valley
Cold cereal: Kashi 7 Whole Grain Puffs

Hot cereal: Arrowhead Mills Instant Plain Oatmeal, Cream of Wheat

Vegan
Meat alternatives: Amy's Kitchen California Veggie Burger, Gardenburger GardenVegan Burger, Tofurky Deli Slices
Vegan cheese: Tofutti, Vegan Essentials, Veggie Slices
Milk alternatives: Almond Breeze Almond Milk, Rice Dream Rice Milk, Soy Dream Unsweetened Soy Milk, Trader Joe's Rice Drink

Vegan and Soy Free
Meat alternatives: Amy's Kitchen California Veggie Burger, Field Roast Deli Slices, Gardenburger GardenVegan Burger
Vegan, soy-free cheese: Vegan Essentials: Vegan rice cheese slices can be purchased online at veganessentials.com. As another option, Vegan Gourmet Cheese alternatives can be purchased at followyourheart.com.
Milk alternatives: Almond Breeze Almond Milk, Rice Dream Rice Milk, Trader Joe's Rice Drink

RESTAURANT RESCUE

Eating away from home is a part of everyday life for most people. Americans eat out for nearly one in every four meals and spend almost half their food budgets on meals away from home.

Whether you're having a business lunch, meeting friends for dinner, or taking the kids out for a special treat, I want you to be able to follow this plan. And it's easy to do. Here are a few key tips for staying on track when dining out.

○ Check out the restaurant menu online. Find some meals that match your favorites in the meal plans. For those restaurants without a Web site, call in advance and ask for the menu to be faxed to you. Also, verify that the restaurant follows a trans-fat-free cooking policy, since trans fats must be eliminated on the *Flat Belly Diet.*

○ At most restaurants, you can order a salad made of leafy greens (about the size of two baseballs) topped with grilled chicken or salmon (about the size of a deck of cards) with balsamic or red wine vinegar and 2 tablespoons of seeds or chopped nuts or 1 tablespoon olive oil. Add a computer mouse–size serving of any one of the following: a whole wheat roll, baked or roasted potato, brown or wild rice, or a starchy vegetable such as beans, peas, or corn.

○ Carry 2 tablespoons of nuts with you in a zip-top bag to supplement meals at restaurants where you might not be able to get a MUFA.

○ Carry a tablespoon with you so that you can measure out nuts or seeds when they are provided by a restaurant.

Order entrées from the lists on the following pages if you're going to one of these popular national chains or look for similar entrées at other restaurants. There is one list for fast-food restaurants and one for sit-down restaurants. The numbers in parentheses are calorie amounts or ranges. MUFAs are listed in boldface.

Fast-Food Restaurant Rescue

Vegetarian Chili, Low Fat, Medium (220). Order the Mixed Nuts and 1 small Fruit Cup (70) and measure 2 tablespoons **nuts** (101) to have on the side.

Total calories: 391

Mediterranean Chicken Salad (290); top with $\frac{1}{4}$ of the Balsamic Vinaigrette dressing (48). This salad comes with olives; include just 10 **olives** (50) on the salad.

Total calories: 388

Spicy Tuna Sandwich; eat $\frac{1}{2}$ sandwich (235). Pair with Garden Salad (70). Order the Mixed Nuts and measure 2 tablespoons **nuts** (101) to have on the side.

Total calories: 406

Split Pea with Ham Soup (250). Order the Mixed Nuts and measure 2 tablespoons **nuts** (101) to have on the side.

Total calories: 351

Order a half-portion Classic Tuna Salad Sandwich (275). Order the Mixed Nuts and measure 2 tablespoons **nuts** (101) to have on the side.

Total calories: 376

Oatmeal, 1 medium cup prepared (210), and 1 small Fruit Cup (70). Order the Mixed Nuts and measure 2 tablespoons **nuts** (101) to add to your oatmeal.

Total calories: 381

Thai Peanut Chicken Salad (240) with $\frac{1}{4}$ of the Thai peanut dressing (60). Order the Mixed Nuts and measure 2 tablespoons **nuts** (101) for the salad or to have on the side.

Total calories: 401

BURGER KING

Tendergrill Garden Salad (220); top with 1/2 packet of light Italian dressing (60). Bring along 2 tablespoons **walnuts** (82) to sprinkle over the salad or to have on the side.

Total calories: 362

CHIPOTLE

Order two 6" Tortilla Wraps (one order comes with three; request two) (180) topped with 1 order Pinto Beans (120), 1 order lettuce (10), and Tomato Salsa (20). Bring along 2 tablespoons **pistachios** (88).

Total calories: 418

DUNKIN' DONUTS

One-half Multigrain Bagel (200), 20-oz medium Latte Lite (160); bring along 2 tablespoons **walnuts** (82).

Total calories: 442

Egg White Turkey Sausage Flatbread Sandwich (280); bring along 2 tablespoons **almonds** (109).

Total calories: 389

EL POLLO LOCO

BRC Burrito, half-portion (194), with side order of Fresh Vegetables, no margarine (35). Bring 2 tablespoons **pumpkin seeds** (148) to have with the vegetables or on the side.

Total calories: 377

Flame-Grilled Skinless Chicken Breast, request skinless (179); with side order of Pinto Beans (138). Bring 2 tablespoons **peanuts** (110).

Total calories: 427

JAMBA JUICE

Order either of the yogurt and fruit blends: Bright Eyed & Blueberry (240) or Sunrise Strawberry (260). Bring along 2 tablespoons **cashews** (100).

Total calories: 340–360

MCDONALD'S

Premium Asian Salad with Grilled Chicken, half-portion (150), with Newman's Own low-fat balsamic vinaigrette (40) and 2 packages of Apple Dippers (70). Request **almonds** on the side and measure out 2 tablespoons (109).

Total calories: 369

Premium Southwest Salad with Grilled Chicken, half-portion (160), with Newman's Own low-fat balsamic vinaigrette (40) and 2 packages of Apple Dippers (70). Request **almonds** on the side and measure out 2 tablespoons (109).

Total calories: 379

PANERA BREAD

Asian Sesame Chicken Salad, half-portion (205); bring along 2 tablespoons **pumpkin seeds** (148).

Total calories: 353

Reduced Fat Wild Blueberry Muffin, half-portion (180), with Fresh Fruit Cup (150). Bring along 2 tablespoons **walnuts** (82).

Total calories: 412

Low-Fat Chicken Noodle Soup (160) with 1 Whole Grain Baguette (140); bring along 2 tablespoons **cashews** (100).

Total calories: 400

Mediterranean Veggie Sandwich, half-portion (305); bring along 2 tablespoons **cashews** (100).

Total calories: 405

Low-Fat Vegetarian Black Bean Soup (250) and Whole Grain Baguette, half-portion (70). Bring along 2 tablespoons **walnuts** (82).

Total calories: 402

Low-Fat Vegetarian Garden Vegetable Soup, 12 ounces (150), with Whole Grain Baguette (140). Bring along 2 tablespoons **almonds** (109).

Total calories: 399

QDOBA MEXICAN GRILL

Mexican Gumbo, half-portion (355). Bring along 2 tablespoons **walnuts** (82).

Total calories: 437

Steak Burrito, half-portion (305). Bring along 2 tablespoons **cashews** (100).

Total calories: 405

SBARRO

One half slice New York Style Thin-Crust Pizza (230) and a large Garden Fresh Salad (70); bring along 2 tablespoons **sunflower seeds** (90) and mix into the salad or have on the side.

Total calories: 390

One half slice New York Style Thin-Crust Fresh Tomato & Basil Pizza (225) and a large Garden Fresh Salad (70); bring along 2 tablespoons **cashews** (100) and mix into the salad or have on the side.

Total calories: 395

Note: For all smoothie options, request no additional enhancers or supplements mixed into the smoothies.

Mangofest, 20 ounces (285); bring along 2 tablespoons **sunflower seeds** (90).

Total calories: 375

Green Tea Tango, 20 ounces (304); bring along 2 tablespoons **sunflower seeds** (90).

Total calories: 394

Island Impact, 20 ounces (312); bring along 2 tablespoons **sunflower seeds** (90).

Total calories: 402

STARBUCKS

Reduced-Fat Blueberry Coffee Cake, half-portion (160), with a tall Nonfat Caffè Latte (100); bring along 2 tablespoons **pumpkin seeds** (148).

Total calories: 408

Plain Bagel, half-portion (155), with a tall Nonfat Caffè Latte (100); bring along 2 tablespoons **pumpkin seeds** (148).

Total calories: 403

SUBWAY

Veggie Delite Sub on whole wheat, 6″ (230), with 2 triangles American cheese (40), a thin layer of mustard (5), and a few shakes of red wine vinegar (0). Ask for **olive oil** on the side and use your tablespoon to measure 1 tablespoon (119), or bring along 2 tablespoons **macadamia nuts** (120) to have on the side.

Total calories: 394–395

Turkey Breast Sub on whole wheat, 6″ (280), with lettuce and 3 tomato slices (5), 2 teaspoons mustard (5), and a few shakes of red wine vinegar (0). Ask for **olive oil** on the side and use your tablespoon to measure 1 tablespoon (119), or bring along 2 tablespoons **macadamia nuts** (120) to have on the side.

Total calories: 409–410

Roast Beef Sub on whole wheat, 6″ (290), with lettuce and 3 tomato slices (5), and a few teaspoons mustard (5), and a few shakes of red wine vinegar (0). Ask for **olive oil** on the side and use your tablespoon to measure 1 tablespoon (119), or bring along 2 tablespoons **macadamia nuts** (120) to have on the side.

Total calories: 419–420

TACO BELL

Fresco Fiesta Chicken Burrito (330) and side of Salsa (15); bring along 2 tablespoons **walnuts** (82).

Total calories: 427

Two Fresco Crunchy Tacos (300) and side of Salsa (15); bring along 2 tablespoons **walnuts** (82).

Total calories: 397

TCBY

Golden Vanilla Yogurt, regular cup (300), topped with 6 strawberries (20); order a side of chopped **walnuts** and measure out 2 tablespoons (82).

Total calories: 402

Chocolate Yogurt, regular cup (275), topped with 6 strawberries (20); order a side of slivered **almonds** and measure out 3 tablespoons (109). (Note that 3 level tablespoons of slivered almonds equal about 2 tablespoons of whole almonds, which is a MUFA serving.)

Total calories: 404

WENDY'S

Mandarin Chicken Salad ordered *without* roasted almonds, crispy noodles, or oriental sesame dressing (180), plus fat-free French dressing (70). Order a side of the Roasted **Almonds** and measure out 2 tablespoons (109).

Total calories: 359

Chicken Caesar Salad ordered *without* supreme Caesar dressing (250), plus ½ packet fat-free French dressing (35). Order a side of Roasted **Almonds** and measure out 2 tablespoons (109).

Total calories: 394

Sit-Down Restaurant Rescue

CHILI'S

Guiltless Cedar Plank Tilapia (199), served with side of Steamed Seasonal Veggies (70). Bring along 2 tablespoons **almonds** (109).

Total calories: 378

Guiltless Grilled Chicken Platter, served with Rice, Corn on the Cob, and Steamed Seasonal Veggies with Parmesan Cheese, half-portion (290). Bring along 2 tablespoons **peanuts** (110).

Total calories: 400

Guiltless Grilled Salmon, served with Black Beans and Steamed Seasonal Veggies with Parmesan Cheese, half-portion (240). Bring along 2 tablespoons **pumpkin seeds** (148).

Total calories: 388

CULVER'S

Stacked Turkey Sandwich, half-portion, no mayo (350). Bring along 2 tablespoons **peanuts** (110).

Total calories: 460

Garden Fresco Salad (235), served with a splash of balsamic vinegar (5) and 3 lemon wedges (16). Bring along 2 tablespoons **pumpkin seeds** (148).

Total calories: 404

Grilled Chicken Breast Sandwich, no butter (344). Bring along 2 tablespoons **walnuts** (82).

Total calories: 426

HOOTERS

Snow Crab Legs, half-portion, no butter (150), with Side Salad, no dressing (60). Request a side of olive oil and vinegar to dress your salad; bring a teaspoon to measure out 1 teaspoon oil (33) and use a splash of vinegar (5). Bring along 2 tablespoons **pumpkin seeds** (148).

Total calories: 396

Steamed Shrimp, no butter or cocktail sauce (230), with Garden Salad, no dressing (115). Request a side of vinegar to dress your salad and use a splash (5). Bring along 2 tablespoons **walnuts** (82).

Total calories: 432

Dozen Raw Oysters, no butter (115), with Garden Salad, no dressing (115). Request a side of olive oil and vinegar to dress your salad; bring a teaspoon to measure out 1 teaspoon oil (33) and use a splash of vinegar (5). Bring along 2 tablespoons **peanuts** (110).

Total calories: 378

Grilled Chicken Garden Salad, no dressing (265). Request a side of olive oil and vinegar to dress your salad; bring a teaspoon to measure out 1 teaspoon oil (33) and use a splash of vinegar (5). Bring along 2 tablespoons **peanuts** (110).

Total calories: 413

MIMI'S CAFE

Low-Fat Fitness Omelet (egg white omelet filled with tomato, mushrooms, and broccoli) and wheat toast, no butter, half-portion (253). Bring along 2 tablespoons **pumpkin seeds** (148).

Total calories: 401

Fresh Roasted Turkey Breast Sandwich on whole wheat, no mayo, with fresh fruit, half-portion (336). Bring along 2 tablespoons **walnuts** (82).

Total calories: 418

Chicken and Fruit, half-portion (213). Bring along 2 tablespoons **pumpkin seeds** (148).

Total calories: 361

OLD SPAGHETTI FACTORY

Spaghetti with Sautéed Mushroom Sauce, half-portion (335). Bring along 2 tablespoons **walnuts** (82).

Total calories: 417

Spaghetti with Marinara Sauce, half-portion (230), with House Salad with Fat Free Honey Mustard dressing (120). Bring along 2 tablespoons **walnuts** (82).

Total calories: 432

PANDA EXPRESS

Mushroom Chicken, steamed (150), with 2 orders of Mixed Vegetables, steamed (180). Bring along 2 tablespoons **cashews** (100).

Total calories: 430

Broccoli Beef, steamed (170), with 2 orders of Mixed Vegetables, steamed (180). Bring along 2 tablespoons **pistachios** (88).

Total calories: 438

Kung Pao Shrimp (210) with Veggie Spring Roll (80). Bring along 2 tablespoons **walnuts** (82).

Total calories: 372

RED LOBSTER

Two Chilled Jumbo Shrimp cocktail appetizers (240) with 2 orders of Steamed Broccoli (90). Bring along 2 tablespoons **walnuts** (82).

Total calories: 412

Grilled Lobster, half-portion (125), and baked potato (190). Order **olive oil** on the side and use your tablespoon to measure 1 tablespoon (119) to drizzle over the potato; sprinkle with black pepper (0).

Total calories: 434

SIZZLER

Grilled Shrimp Skewers with Rice Pilaf, half portion (260). Bring along 2 tablespoons **cashews** (120).

Total calories: 380

BEST MEAL CHOICES

If you're eating out at a restaurant that's not listed with our Restaurant Rescue, follow these guidelines to build a *Flat Belly Diet* meal. Bring along a tablespoon for all outings; this will help you measure out your MUFA and be sure that you are sticking to the *Flat Belly Diet* calorie guidelines. In some cases, you won't be able to find a MUFA, so bring along 2 tablespoons of nuts or seeds in a zip-top bag. A specific type of nuts or seeds that will complement your meal is listed, but feel free to substitute those that you have already packed or like best.

At Different Types of Restaurants

Note: Chinese restaurants will let you order most dishes steamed. Most tea cups in a Chinese restaurant are about $\frac{1}{2}$ cup, so you can use this to measure out your portions.

Order steamed mixed vegetables and have 2 cups (100). Have $\frac{1}{2}$ cup steamed brown rice (if this is not available, select white rice) (80). Have 1 cup hot-and-sour soup or wonton soup (110). Order a side of **cashews** and measure out 2 tablespoons (100); mix them with your vegetables and rice or have on the side.

Total calories: 390

Order 6 steamed vegetable dumplings (150). Have 1 cup steamed brown rice (if this is not available, select white rice) (160). Order a side of **cashews** and measure out 2 tablespoons (100); sprinkle them over your vegetable dumplings and rice or have on the side.

Total calories: 410

Order steamed mixed vegetables with shrimp and have 2 cups (200). Have $\frac{1}{2}$ cup steamed brown rice (if this is not available, select white rice) (80). Order a side of **cashews** and measure out 2 tablespoons (100); mix them with your vegetables and rice or have on the side.

Total calories: 380

Order a sandwich made of 2 slices whole wheat bread (160), 4 ounces deli sliced turkey (140), 3 tomato slices (5), a handful of shredded lettuce (0), 1 packet of mustard (5), and 10 black or green **olives** (50). Have 1 medium apple (60).

Total calories: 420

Order 1 small salad (35), no dressing, with 6 tomato slices (10), 10 cucumber slices (10), 3 ounces grilled chicken (110), and a splash of balsamic vinegar (5). Order **olive oil** on the side and use your tablespoon to measure 1 tablespoon (119). Have 1 slice whole wheat bread on the side (80).

Total calories: 369

AN ITALIAN TRATTORIA

Order cooked pasta, preferably whole wheat, and have 1 cup (about the size of a baseball) (175). Measure out 1 tablespoon **olive oil** (119). Top your pasta with half of the oil plus 1 tablespoon grated Parmesan cheese (22) and ground black pepper (0). Have a side salad (35); mix the other half of the oil with a splash of vinegar (5) to make a salad dressing. Have $3/4$ cup minestrone soup (80) *or* a 2-ounce portion (the size of 2 matchbooks) of salmon that's baked or broiled with no added oil (90).

Total calories: 436–446

A JAPANESE SUSHI BAR

Note: Most tea cups in a Japanese restaurant are about $1/2$ cup, so you can use this to measure out your portions. You can also use visual cues to stay on track; 1 cup steamed brown rice is about the size of a baseball.

Order tuna roll sushi and have 5 pieces (154). Have 1 cup steamed brown rice (if this is not available, select white rice) (160). Bring along 2 tablespoons **cashews** (100).

Total calories: 414

Order cucumber roll sushi and have 6 pieces (136). Have 1 cup steamed brown rice (if this is not available, select white rice) (160). Bring along 2 tablespoons **cashews** (100).

Total calories: 396

Order 1 slice cheese pizza from a large pie (272). Have a side salad (35) dressed with a splash of vinegar (5). Bring along 2 tablespoons **pine nuts** (113).

Total calories: 425

Order grilled steak and have 3 ounces (about the size of a deck of cards) (160). Have 1 cup green beans, carrots, or other vegetable (about the size of a baseball) (50) and $\frac{1}{2}$ small baked potato (64). Order a side of **olive oil** and measure out 1 tablespoon (119) to drizzle over the vegetables.

Total calories: 393

Order grilled chicken steak and have 3 ounces (about the size of a deck of cards) (160). Have 1 cup green beans, carrots, or other vegetable (about the size of a baseball) (50). Order a side of **olive oil** and measure out 1 tablespoon (119) to drizzle over the vegetables. Have 1 small dinner roll, white or whole wheat (80).

Total calories: 409

At Events and Entertainment Venues

Before you leave for the movie theater, ball game, carnival, theme park, or other destinations, pack your own *Flat Belly Diet* Snack Pack. Always include one small piece of fruit and 2 tablespoons of nuts or seeds packed in a zip-top bag. Also included here are some of the best choices you can make with what you might find available. The good news? Even these venues are beginning to offer healthier choices, including fresh fruit and nuts, thanks to demand from smart eaters like you!

Have 1 cup (a little more than half the package) Cracker Jack original caramel-coated popcorn (240). Bring 1 piece of fruit, like a small apple or medium orange (62), and 2 tablespoons **peanuts** (110).

Total calories: 412

Have 1 small hamburger (254). Bring 1 piece of fruit, like a small apple or medium orange (62), and 2 tablespoons **walnuts** (82).

Total calories: 398

Order a soft pretzel (340) drizzled with 1 packet of mustard (5). Bring along 2 tablespoons **walnuts** (82).

Total calories: 427

Order a beef hot dog on a bun and have half (143) with 1 packet of ketchup (15). Bring 1 piece of fruit, like a small apple or medium orange (62), and 2 tablespoons **pumpkin seeds** (148).

Total calories: 368

Order corn tortilla chips and have about 16 chips (176). Bring 1 piece of fruit, like a small apple or medium orange (62), and 2 tablespoons **peanuts** (110).

Total calories: 348

A CARNIVAL OR STREET FAIR

Order popcorn (air popped, without butter) and have 6 cups (about half of what you would find in a typical bag of microwave popcorn) (180). Bring 1 piece of fruit, like a small apple or medium orange (62), and 2 tablespoons **peanuts** (110).

Total calories: 352

Order a soft pretzel and have half (170). Bring along $1/4$ cup **semisweet or dark chocolate chips** (207).

Total calories: 377

Order corn tortilla chips and have about 16 chips (176).
Bring 1 piece of fruit, like a small apple or medium orange
(62), and 2 tablespoons **pumpkin seeds** (148).

Total calories: 386

Note: Consider taking along your snacks instead of purchasing food at the theater. You'll save money and stay the course with your diet. Here are some *Flat Belly Diet*–approved suggestions.

Make Your Own Trail Mix 1: Combine 1 small (1.5-ounce)
box raisins (130), 2 tablespoons **peanuts** (110), and 20
unsalted mini pretzels (110).

Total calories: 350

Make Your Own Trail Mix 2: Combine ¼ cup **semisweet or
dark chocolate chips** (207), 1 small (1.5-ounce) box raisins
(130), and 10 unsalted mini pretzels (55).

Total calories: 392

Bring 6 cups air-popped popcorn without butter (about
half of what you would find in a typical bag of microwave
popcorn) (180) and ¼ cup **semisweet or dark chocolate
chips** (207).

Total calories: 387

Order 1 soft pretzel (340) with 1 packet of mustard (5);
bring along 2 tablespoons **walnuts** (82).

Total calories: 427

Order 1 small Dippin' Dots low-fat fudge ice cream (150).
Bring 1 piece of fruit, like a small apple or medium orange
(62), and ¼ cup **semisweet or dark chocolate chips** (207)
to top your ice cream or to have on the side.

Total calories: 419

Order a beef hot dog on a bun and have half (143) with 1 packet of ketchup (15). Bring 1 piece of fruit, like a small apple or medium orange (62), and ¼ cup **semisweet or dark chocolate chips** (207).

Total calories: 427

Order 1 slice cheese pizza from a large pie (272) and 1 side salad (35) with a splash of vinegar (5). Bring along 2 tablespoons **cashews** (100).

Total calories: 412

Order 1 small hamburger (254). Bring 1 piece of fruit, like a small apple or medium orange (62), and 2 tablespoons **walnuts** (82).

Total calories: 398

A VENDING MACHINE

Get 2 Nature Valley Crunchy Granola Bars, oats & honey flavor (180). Bring 1 piece of fruit, like a small apple or medium orange (62), and 2 tablespoons **pumpkin seeds** (148).

Total calories: 390

Get Baked Lay's Original Potato Crisps, original flavor, and have 2 ounces or 22 chips (220). Bring 1 piece of fruit, like a small apple or medium orange (62), and 2 tablespoons **peanuts** (110).

Total calories: 392

Get Animal Crackers, regular flavor, and have 16 crackers (120) *or* get 100-calorie pack snacks (any variety with 3 grams or less saturated fat) (100). Bring 1 piece of fruit, like a small apple or medium orange (62), and ¼ cup **semisweet or dark chocolate chips** (207).

Total calories: 369–389

CONCLUSION

Losing belly fat helps your health but also gives you plenty of confidence. I know what it's like to work lots of hours and not find the time to shop for healthy foods, plan take-along meals and snacks, and continue to eat healthfully even while traveling. Celebrations, vacations, and life can get in the way sometimes. But you can regain control over what you put in your mouth with this plan. Here you have the tools you need to follow the *Flat Belly Diet consistently* and make a flatter belly a reality.

Follow the *Flat Belly Diet* for as long as it takes for you to reach your goal weight. The 1,600-calorie plan was calculated to help you get to, and then also maintain, your goal weight. Diets shouldn't require a calorie readjustment for maintenance. The problem with most diets is that giving you fewer calories than it takes to support your healthy weight goal (then increasing once you get there) can cause not only a loss of body fat but also a loss of muscle mass and bone density, plus a weaker immune system. For most women, 1,600 calories provides enough calories to support your ideal or target weight—that means once you reach that weight, the plan will allow you to maintain it. If you continue to lose weight, beyond your goal weight, add back one-half to one snack until you begin to maintain your weight.

This plan is less about achieving a slim body than it is about creating a healthy life. The MUFAs and other healthful foods on the plan are just the fuel you need to fight disease and maintain your healthiest body ever.

COMMON CONVERSIONS

TEASPOON (TSP)	TABLESPOON (TBSP)	CUPS	PINT/QUART/GALLON	FLUID OUNCE (OZ)	MILLILITER
1 tsp	$\frac{1}{3}$ Tbsp				5 ml
3 tsp	1 Tbsp	$\frac{1}{16}$ cup		0.5 oz	15 ml
6 tsp	2 Tbsp	$\frac{1}{8}$ cup		1 oz	30 ml
12 tsp	4 Tbsp	$\frac{1}{4}$ cup		2 oz	60 ml
16 tsp	$5\frac{1}{3}$ Tbsp	$\frac{1}{3}$ cup		2.5 oz	75 ml
24 tsp	8 Tbsp	$\frac{1}{2}$ cup		4 oz	125 ml
32 tsp	$10\frac{2}{3}$ Tbsp	$\frac{2}{3}$ cup		5 oz	150 ml
36 tsp	12 Tbsp	$\frac{3}{4}$ cup		6 oz	175 ml
48 tsp	16 Tbsp	1 cup	$\frac{1}{2}$ pint	8 oz	237 ml
		2 cups	1 pint	16 oz	473 ml
		3 cups		24 oz	710 ml
		4 cups	1 quart	32 oz	946 ml
		8 cups	$\frac{1}{2}$ gallon	64 oz	
		16 cups	1 gallon	128 oz	

YOUR MUFA SERVING CHART

FOOD	SERVING	CALORIES
OILS		
Canola oil	1 Tbsp	124
Flaxseed oil (cold-pressed organic)	1 Tbsp	120
Olive oil	1 Tbsp	119
Peanut oil	1 Tbsp	119
Pesto sauce	1 Tbsp	80
Safflower oil (high oleic)	1 Tbsp	120
Sesame or soybean oil	1 Tbsp	120
Sunflower oil (high oleic)	1 Tbsp	120
Walnut oil	1 Tbsp	120
NUTS, LEGUMES, AND SEEDS		
Almonds	2 Tbsp	109
Almond butter	2 Tbsp	200
Brazil nuts	2 Tbsp	110
Cashews	2 Tbsp	100
Cashew butter	2 Tbsp	190
Edamame (soybeans), shelled and boiled	1 cup	298
Hazelnuts	2 Tbsp	110
Macadamia nuts	2 Tbsp	120
Peanuts	2 Tbsp	110
Peanut butter (natural), crunchy	2 Tbsp	188
Peanut butter (natural), smooth	2 Tbsp	188

FOOD	SERVING	CALORIES
Pecans	2 Tbsp	90
Pine nuts	2 Tbsp	113
Pistachios	2 Tbsp	88
Pumpkin seeds	2 Tbsp	148
Sunflower seeds	2 Tbsp	90
Sunflower seed butter	2 Tbsp	190
Tahini (sesame seed paste)	2 Tbsp	178
Walnuts	2 Tbsp	82

AVOCADOS

Avocado, California (Hass)	¼ cup	96
Avocado, Florida	¼ cup	69

OLIVES

Black olive tapenade	2 Tbsp	88
Green olive tapenade	2 Tbsp	54
Green or black olives	10 large	50

DARK CHOCOLATE

Semisweet or dark chocolate chips	¼ cup	207

EAT THESE FOODS REGULARLY
LEAN PROTEIN

FOOD	SERVING SIZE	CALORIES
BEANS AND LEGUMES		

Note: When using canned beans, rinse in a colander for 2 to 3 minutes under cool running water to remove up to one-third of the sodium.

FOOD	SERVING SIZE	CALORIES
Adzuki beans, cooked	½ cup	147
Alfalfa sprouts	½ cup	5
Baked beans, homemade with brown sugar	⅓ cup	126
Baked beans, vegetarian	⅓ cup	113
Baked beans, with beef or pork	⅓ cup	113
Bean sprouts, kidney	½ cup	30
Bean sprouts, mung	½ cup	13
Black-eyed peas (cowpeas), cooked	½ cup	90
Black turtle beans, cooked	½ cup	120
Broad beans (fava beans), cooked	½ cup	62
Butter beans (lima), cooked	½ cup	105
Butter beans (lima), raw	½ cup	88
Cannellini beans, cooked	½ cup	100
Chickpeas (garbanzo beans), cooked	½ cup	134
Chili, vegetarian, canned	½ cup	103
Chili, with meat, low-fat, canned	½ cup	154
Cranberry beans, cooked	½ cup	120
Edamame (soybeans), unshelled, cooked	½ cup	100
Great Northern beans, cooked	½ cup	104
Green beans, cooked	½ cup	114
Green beans, raw	3 oz	30

FOOD	SERVING SIZE	CALORIES
Kidney beans, red, cooked	½ cup	110
Lentils, brown, cooked	½ cup	115
Mung beans, cooked	½ cup	106
Navy beans, cooked	½ cup	127
Pinto beans, cooked	½ cup	122
Refried beans, fat-free, canned	½ cup	45
Refried beans, traditional, canned	½ cup	100
Split peas, cooked	½ cup	115
BEEF AND PORK		
Beef, bottom round, trimmed, boneless, braised	3 oz	108
Beef, chuck roast, lean, braised	3 oz	179
Beef, eye round, lean, roasted	3 oz	138
Beef, filet mignon, lean, broiled	3 oz	179
Beef, flank steak, lean, broiled	4 oz	187
Beef, steak, top sirloin, lean, broiled	3 oz	166
Beef, tip sirloin, lean, roasted	3 oz	152
Canadian bacon, grilled	1 oz	52
Ham, low-sodium, 96% fat-free	1 oz	31
Pork, chop, center-cut, roasted	4 oz	187
Pork tenderloin, roasted	3 oz	115
EGGS		
Eggs	1 large	75
Egg white	¼ cup	29

FOOD	SERVING SIZE	CALORIES
POULTRY		
Chicken breast, roasted	3 oz	140
Chicken, drumstick, without skin, cooked	3 oz	146
Chicken, ground, without skin, cooked	3 oz	173
Chicken, thigh, boneless, without skin, cooked	3 oz	166
Turkey burger, 90% lean, cooked	3 oz	170
Turkey, deli	2 oz	50
Turkey, drumstick, without skin, cooked	3 oz	159
Turkey pepperoni, sliced	1 oz	69
Turkey, roasted	3 oz	162
Turkey sausage, Italian, lean, cooked	2 oz	95
SEAFOOD		
Cod, Atlantic, baked	3 oz	89
Crab, Alaskan, king crab leg, steamed	3 oz	83
Crab, blue, cooked	3 oz	101
Crab, imitation (surimi)	3 oz	87
Flounder, baked	3 oz	99
Grouper, baked	3 oz	100
Halibut, baked	3 oz	119
Lobster, cooked	3 oz	81
Mahi mahi, baked	3 oz	93
Salmon, Alaskan chinook, smoked, canned	3 oz	128
Salmon, wild, canned, drained	3 oz	135
Shrimp, broiled	4 oz	120
Swordfish, baked	3 oz	132
Tilapia, baked or broiled	3 oz	109
Tuna, chunk light, packed in water	3 oz	120
Tuna, yellowfin, baked	3 oz	118

FOOD	SERVING SIZE	CALORIES
Cheddar cheese, reduced-fat, shredded	¼ cup	81
Cottage cheese, fat-free	½ cup	90
Feta cheese, crumbled	1 tablespoon	40
Milk, fat-free	1 cup	80
Milk, 1% low-fat	1 cup	102
Parmesan cheese, grated	1 tablespoon	21
Provolone cheese, reduced-fat	1 oz	77
Rice milk, plain, enriched	1 cup	130
Ricotta cheese, fat-free	¼ cup	50
Sour cream, fat-free	1 tablespoon	15
Soy milk, plain, unsweetened	1 cup	80
Yogurt, fat-free Greek-style	½ cup	56
Yogurt, fat-free vanilla	½ cup	103

FRUITS AND VEGETABLES

FOOD	SERVING SIZE	CALORIES
FRUIT		
Apple	1 medium	95
Applesauce, unsweetened, canned	⅓ cup	33
Apricot	1 medium	17
Apricot, dried	6 pieces	60
Banana	1 small (6")	90
Blackberries	1 cup	62
Blueberries	½ cup	40
Cantaloupe, balled	1 cup	60
Cantaloupe, wedged	⅛ large	35
Cherries, sweet	½ cup	50

FOOD	SERVING SIZE	CALORIES
Clementine	1 medium	40
Date, medjool, pitted	1 medium	66
Fig	1 large	47
Grapefruit	½ medium	60
Grapes, green or red	1 cup	104
Guava	1 medium	61
Honeydew, balled	1 cup	64
Honeydew, wedged	⅛ medium	58
Kiwifruit (Chinese gooseberry), peeled	1 medium	46
Mandarin oranges, canned	½ cup	80
Mango, sliced	1 cup	120
Nectarine	1 medium	70
Orange	1 medium	62
Papaya, cubed	1 cup	55
Peach	1 medium	38
Pear	1 medium	104
Pineapple, sliced	1 cup	100
Pineapple, tidbits	½ cup or 4 oz	60
Plum	1 (2⅛")	30
Plum, sliced	½ cup	47
Pomegranate	½ medium	53
Pomelo, sectioned	½ cup	36
Raspberries, red	1 cup	64
Rhubarb, diced	1 cup	26
Star fruit (carambola)	1 medium	28
Tangerine	1 medium	50
Watermelon, chopped	1 cup	45

FOOD	SERVING SIZE	CALORIES
VEGETABLES		
Artichoke	1 medium	60
Artichoke hearts, cooked, drained	½ cup	42
Arugula (rocket)	4 oz	28
Asparagus, cooked	1 cup	30
Beets, cooked	½ cup	37
Beets, pickled, whole, canned	½ cup	65
Bell pepper, sliced	1 cup	46
Bok choy, cooked, drained	1 cup	20
Broccoli, florets	1 cup	20
Broccoli rabe, cooked	1 cup	28
Brussels sprouts, cooked	1 cup	65
Cabbage	¼ medium head	54
Carrot	1 medium	25
Carrots, cooked, drained	½ cup	27
Cauliflower	¼ large head	53
Cauliflower, florets, cooked	1 cup	39
Celery	1 medium stalk	9
Celery, chopped	1 cup	17
Cherry tomatoes, red	1 cup	27
Collard greens, chopped, cooked, drained	1 cup	49
Cucumber	1 (8")	45
Eggplant, cubed, cooked, drained	1 cup	35
Fennel bulb, sliced	1 cup	27
Garlic	1 clove	4
Garlic, chopped	1 tsp	4
Ginger, fresh, grated	1 Tbsp	5
Green beans, fresh	1 cup	35
Kale, curly, cooked	1 cup	36
Lettuce, bibb	1 (5") head	21

FOOD	SERVING SIZE	CALORIES
Lettuce, mixed baby	2 cups	15
Lettuce, romaine, chopped	1 cup	8
Mushrooms, portobello	2 oz	15
Mushrooms, portobello, grilled	3 oz	29
Onion, red, chopped	½ cup	34
Onion, red or yellow	1 medium	46
Onion, red or yellow, sliced	1 large slice	16
Onion, yellow, chopped	½ cup	34
Pepper, ancho, dried	1 medium	47
Sauerkraut, low-sodium, canned	1 cup	31
Scallion, top and bulb, chopped	½ cup	16
Shallots, chopped	¼ cup	29
Spaghetti squash, baked	1 cup	42
Spinach, baby	1 cup	8
Spinach, cooked	1 cup	41
Squash, summer, raw	1 medium	31
Squash, summer, sliced, cooked	1 cup	36
Swiss chard, chopped, cooked, drained	1 cup	35
Tomatillo	1 medium	11
Tomatillo, chopped	½ cup	21
Tomato, red grape	1 cup	30
Tomato, plum	1 medium	12
Tomato, red	1 medium	35
Tomato, red, chopped	½ cup	19
Tomato, red, crushed, canned	½ cup	39
Tomato, red, sliced	1 slice	6
Tomato paste	1 tablespoon	13
Zucchini	1 medium	35
Zucchini, sliced, steamed	1 cup	25

GRAINS AND STARCHY VEGETABLES

FOOD	SERVING SIZE	CALORIES
BREAD AND CRACKERS		
Bagel, whole grain	1 oz	75
Bread, French, whole grain	1 slice (1 oz)	90
Bread, pita, whole wheat	½ of 6″ pita	70
Bread, whole wheat	1 slice (1 oz)	80
Bread crumbs, dry	1 oz	112
Bun, hamburger, whole grain	1 bun (1 oz)	90
Cracker, crispbread, rye	¾ oz	78
Cracker, small whole wheat	4 crackers	72
English muffin, whole wheat	About 2.4 oz or 1 muffin	140
Roll, dinner, whole wheat	1 roll (1 oz)	77
PASTA AND GRAINS		
Note: For most pasta shapes, 1 ounce of dry pasta makes approximately ½ cup cooked.		
Barley, pearled, cooked	¼ cup	48
Bulgur, cooked	⅓ cup	50
Chips, baked	1 oz	120
Couscous, whole wheat, cooked	½ cup	108
Oats, rolled, dry	½ cup	150
Pasta or spaghetti, any shape, gluten-free, cooked	½ cup	100
Pasta or spaghetti, any shape, whole wheat, cooked	½ cup	87
Pilaf, 7-grain cooked	¼ cup	85
Quinoa, cooked	¼ cup	81
Rice, basmati, cooked	½ cup	102
Rice, brown, medium grain, cooked	½ cup	109
Rice, wild, cooked	½ cup	83

FOOD	SERVING SIZE	CALORIES
Soba noodles, cooked	1 cup	113
Tortilla, corn	6"	57
Tortilla chips, multigrain, baked	½ oz	60

Corn, sweet white or yellow	1 large ear	123
Corn, sweet white or yellow	½ cup	66
Peas, cooked	½ cup	62
Plantain	¼ medium	55
Potato, baked, with skin	1 medium	162
Potato, russet, baked, with skin	1 medium	160
Potatoes, baby, roasted	1 cup	100
Potatoes, new, cooked	3 oz	54
Squash, acorn, cooked, mashed	½ cup	42
Squash, acorn, cubed, baked	½ cup	57
Squash, butternut, cubed, baked	1 cup	82
Sweet potato, baked, without skin	1 medium	103
Sweet potato, cooked, mashed	½ cup	125

OTHER

FOOD	SERVING SIZE	CALORIES
SWEETENERS AND CONDIMENTS		
Apple butter	1 Tbsp	29
Barbecue sauce	1 Tbsp	12
Fruit spread, any flavor	1 Tbsp	40
Honey	1 tsp	30
Horseradish sauce	1 Tbsp	30
Ketchup	1 Tbsp	16
Mayonnaise, canola	1 Tbsp	100

FOOD	SERVING SIZE	CALORIES
Mustard	1 Tbsp	10
Mustard, Dijon, coarse-grain	1 Tbsp	15
Salsa, medium	2 Tbsp	9
Soy sauce	1 Tbsp	11
Vinegar, balsamic or red wine	1 Tbsp	10
Worcestershire sauce	1 Tbsp	11

BEVERAGES

FOOD	SERVING SIZE	CALORIES
Almond milk, Almond Breeze, unsweetened, original, vanilla, or chocolate	1 cup	40–45
Cappuccino, with low-fat milk	1 cup	73
Chai, with soy milk	1 cup	130
Coffee, iced latte, with fat-free milk	1 cup	47
Iced tea, unsweetened	1 cup	0
Tomato-vegetable juice, low-sodium	1 cup	53

If you don't like plain water, add any of the following juices once or twice per day to plain water for flavor. One ounce of juice is 2 tablespoons or $1/8$ cup. For the best results on the *Flat Belly Diet* plan, please account for the juice calories in your meal plan and please select 100 percent juice only.

FOOD	SERVING SIZE	CALORIES
Apple juice	1 oz	14
Cherry juice	1 oz	19
Cranberry juice	1 oz	17
Grape juice	1 oz	19
Mango juice	1 oz	18
Orange juice	1 oz	14
Pineapple juice	1 oz	16
Pomegranate juice	1 oz	20
Prune juice	1 oz	22
Tangerine juice	1 oz	18

EAT THESE FOODS SPARINGLY

You can include these foods in your meals up to three times per week. For full-fat cheese, be sure to account for the saturated fat in your meal so you don't go over 4 grams of saturated fat per meal. Some full-fat cheeses have up to 6 grams of saturated fat per 1-ounce slice, so check your nutrition facts label.

FOOD	SERVING SIZE	CALORIES
PROTEIN		
Cheese, sliced, full-fat	1 oz or 1 slice	100–120
Cottage cheese, 2% reduced-fat	$\frac{1}{2}$ cup	102
DAIRY		
Milk, 2% reduced-fat	1 cup	122
GRAINS		
Bread or rolls, white flour	1 oz	75
Crackers, white flour	$\frac{1}{2}$ oz	61
Hominy, white, canned	$\frac{1}{2}$ cup	59
Pasta, semolina, cooked	$\frac{1}{2}$ cup	102
Pasta, white flour, cooked	$\frac{1}{2}$ cup	95
Rice, white, cooked	$\frac{1}{2}$ cup	121
OTHER		
Sugar, granulated	1 tsp	16

INDEX

The hottest diet in America!

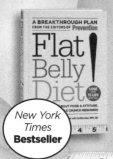

A breakthrough plan from the editors of PREVENTION, *Flat Belly Diet!* gives you all the tips and moves you need to eliminate belly bulge—no crunches required! *Flat Belly Diet!* gives you the skinny on belly fat—how it got there (easily), how it affects your health (poorly), and how eating the right foods can help you get rid of it (finally!). Plus, you'll learn how to master the mind-belly connection, eliminate self-sabotage, conquer emotional eating, and develop a slimmer, leaner waistline. Best of all, *Flat Belly Diet!* makes it all so, so simple with easy-to-follow instructions, quick-fix meal plans, and delicious recipes.

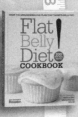

The *Flat Belly Diet! Cookbook* is for the food-lover in you, with 200 all-new seriously tasty recipes, a guide to making your own *Flat Belly Diet!*-friendly meals from scratch, and tips on buying and preparing your key foods.

The *Flat Belly Diet! Journal* is your essential tool to track what you eat and strengthen your daily commitment to lifelong health and vitality.

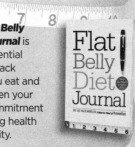

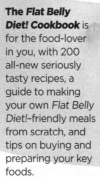

The Flat Belly Workout Express Belly Blast DVD is a combination cardio, toning, and yoga program that will help you burn fat, boost metabolism, and beat stress—the hidden cause of belly flab.

The Flat Belly Workout Walk Off Belly Fat DVD is an easy-to-follow 25-minute indoor workout that combines simple walking moves with torso-toning exercises.

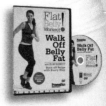

201126601

Lose up to 15 pounds in 32 days with this breakthrough plan! Visit FLATBELLYDIET.COM and order your copies today